YOUR COMPLETE GUIDE TO

Aromatherapy

YOUR NATURAL RESOURCE TO ESSENTIAL OILS FOR WEIGHT-LOSS, STRESS, ANTI-AGING AND SO MUCH MORE!

Learn How To Create Your Own Recipes for Your Child, Pet and Yourself! Easy Reference Charts!

B.THOMAS-SMITH

Your Complete Guide to Aromatherapy

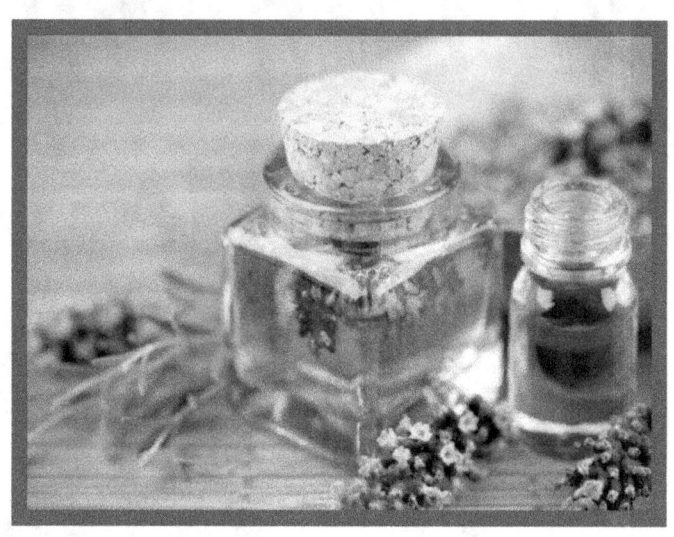

Your Natural Resource to Essential Oils for Weight Loss, Stress, Anti-Aging and Much More

"Believe with all of your heart that you will do what you were made to do."
Orison Swett Marden

Thank you kindly for purchasing this Aromatherapy book and I thank you from the bottom of my heart for helping me to make in a difference in other's lives. Your thoughtful and positive reviews are greatly appreciated.

My main focus for this book is what I hope to accomplish with it (and the others following this). Making a difference is something I am driven to do and this is a way I know I can accomplish that, my sincere thanks to all of you who will help me accomplish my dream.

20% of the proceeds are going to be donated to the Cancer Society as that is what ended up taking my dad's life on November 25th, 2012.

Dedication

This book is first dedicated to God. Thank you for all your blessings & favours.

To Joan, for giving us these great recipes...you are still sadly missed.

To my dad who passed away in November. Dad I love & miss you terribly. There isn't a moment that goes by where I wish that I could talk to you, hear your voice and give you a hug. Thank you for giving me your artistic talent, your encouragement and support for everything I did.

Last but not least, this is also dedicated to my husband Michael and my fur babies (Keysha, Blue, Tess, Shamrock & Gabrielle). Thank you for your love, strength and support, I truly couldn't have made it without you. Love you always!

Table of Contents

Introduction

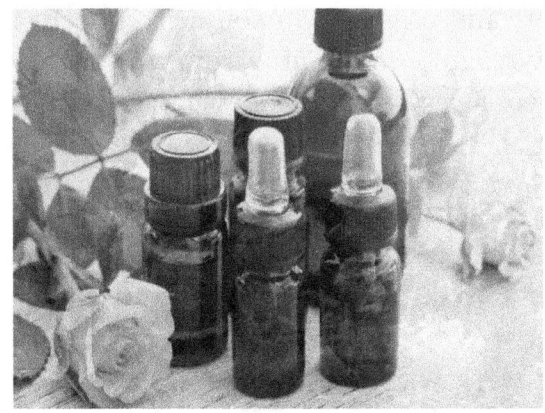

Thank you for downloading *Your Complete Guide to Aromatherapy.*

Through this book you are about to embark on a wonderful quest - one that's filled with discovery, fun facts and easy to procure solution for everyday ailments in your household.

Herbs, flowers, leaves, nuts, seeds, roots - nature is filled with various types of plant sources that have been of immeasurable value to us for centuries. Since the dawn of civilization, man has turned to these humble yet mighty agents of nourishment, medication, and therapy. We may have strayed away from the world of natural therapy since the advent of technological means, but nature today is finding its footing again as an effective means of treatment.

Aromatherapy is an art form - a science really - that focuses on the essences from these natural plant sources for a means of therapy and medication. Through essential oils extracted from flowers, plants and other green sources, you can find solutions to nearly any plaguing ailment - from aches and pains, to bad breath, to even cures for the mold in your home! How to work with these essences of nature is what this book is about.

Through the first chapter, you will dive into the world of aromatherapy with a brief introduction on the essential oils. You will learn more about their structure, nature and compatibility with your body. We will then move on to learning more about how you can work with these essences from nature. From the processes of extraction, to the blends that can be created, you will have a good understanding of aromatherapy by this point.

Once you are armed with information, we will step into the next chapter that involves setting up your aromatherapy kit. Packed with information on the right way to procure your ingredients to safety guidelines to be aware of, this chapter helps you gain a well-rounded perspective on the effects of aromatherapy.

The next chapter shows you practical blends that cure everyday ailments. Through chapter three, you will find oil blends to help relieve ailments like coughs, headaches and stomach aches, first-aid emergencies like cuts, wounds and bruises. You will also learn how to treat such ailments as halitosis, ear infections and dizzy spells.

Chapters four and five focus on therapy for your cosmetic as well as mental needs. You will find oil blends for your facial massages, and daily cleansing routines, along with shampoo remedies, and blends that address menstrual issues. You will also find blends that help relieve symptoms of stress, tension and help rejuvenate you.

Finally, chapter six focuses on your home and hearth, by giving you blends to freshen up the kitchen, bathroom and living spaces, along with cures for your pets and the garden areas.

So what are you waiting for? The world of aromatherapy beckons with its many secrets - let's begin unraveling them one at a time!

Chapter 1: Enter the World of Aromatherapy

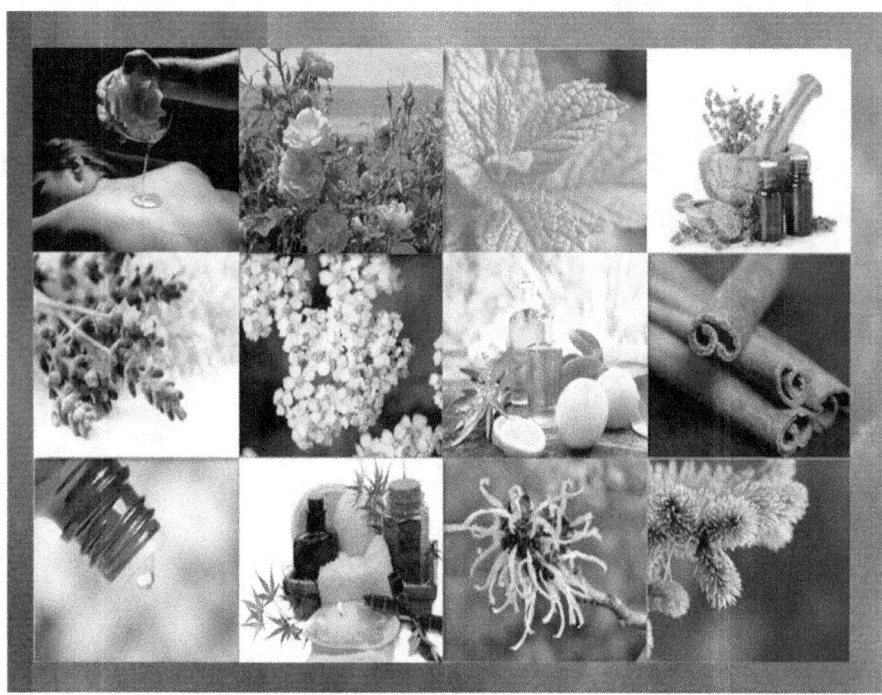

To kick things off, let's begin with a closer look at the world of Aromatherapy. This world is, in fact, so diverse and complex, that a few pages will not do it sufficient justice. There are about 300 essential oils in today's world that can be used to cure a variety of ailments - from blood pressure and digestion troubles, to relieving stress, improving your moods and calming your nerves down. Through this chapter, I will help you try and navigate your first steps in this fascinating world.

Aromatherapy is the science that employs the use of essential oils in different methods to help and alleviate different physical and mental discomforts. Through this chapter, you will first gain a better understanding on the nature of essential oils - how they are sourced and extracted and how they can be used. You will also learn a little about the chemistry behind essential oils, along with their benefits and uses. With this information, you will be ready to start building your aromatherapy kit to suit your personal needs.

Understanding Essential Oils

Simply put, essential oils are nothing but the "essences" derived from various plant sources in nature. The purpose of this extracted oil is to be of some therapeutic benefit, be it physical, mental or emotional. Before you begin procuring and blending these oils to create your aromatherapy kit, it helps to have a broader understanding of the nature and use of these oils.

Sources of Essential Oils

Essential oils are extracted from natural plant sources such as trees, flowers, herbs, shrubs and grasses. This does not mean that every root, leaf or shrub has highly medicinal properties. Essential oils are only effective when derived from certain species of plants that have been cultivated under the right conditions, and have been extracted by the right methods.

In the plant itself, the oil may be found in various locations, within cell pockets created specifically for oil storage. Therefore, you may extract geranium from the leaves and stalks of the plant, but will need to extract ginger oil from the root-structured stems of the plant. Essential oils like mandarin, lemon and lime are extracted from the peels of the fruit, while oils such as cumin are derived from the seeds.

Methods of Use

While many forms of treatment for everyday ailments can be

taken orally, aromatherapy is distinctive in this regard. Essential oils are most beneficial to you when they are taken externally, instead of internally. Surprising as this may be, essential oils are most effective when they are either applied to your skin or inhaled.

This is because ingesting an essential oil brings it into contact with the digestive juices in your system. These highly toxic juices react with the oils, altering their chemical structure. Since essential oils depend on their chemical structure for their therapeutic properties, any altering makes them useless to you.

The most effective ways to use essential oils in treatment and therapy is in the form of massage oils, compresses, body baths, foot soaks, hair rinses or even lotions and tinctures.

Effective ways to inhale essential oils in therapy include steam inhalation treatments, tissue inhalation, perfumes and sprays for the room.

Means of Extraction

Not all plants have the same cellular structure, texture or even appearance. Due to their individual natures, we cannot use just one method to extract their oil in the correct way. The distinctive chemical structures of each plant require the extraction process to be tailored in a way that does not damage its potency or effects.

The most commonly used methods of essential oil extraction are known as Steam Distillation. Methods such as Enfleurage are usually used to extract oils from flowers. Other common methods used include Maceration, Expression and Solvent Extraction, though many other means to successfully extract oils are being devised by the health industry.

Furthermore, the individual nature of plants also means that you don't derive the same amount of oil from the same quantity of every source. Therefore, while you can extract up to 3 pounds of lavender with 100 pounds of lavender flowers, you will only get an ounce of oil from about 60,000 rose blossoms!

The potency of the oil extracted also depends greatly on other conditions, such as the time of extraction, and the age of the plant during extraction. So your jasmine flowers will only yield high-quality essential oil if they are hand-picked before sunrise on the first day that the petal open up and bloom. And even then, you will need to hand-pick 4 million jasmine blossoms to get 1 pound of oil! Sandalwood, on the other hand, will only yield highly potent oil once they are thirty years old and have reached at least thirty feet in height.

Availability of Essential Oils

The process of cultivating and then extracting essential oils from their natural sources is a complicated and drawn-out one. The source plants rely on factors such as the right soil, climate, altitude, water and sunlight to yield potent oil. Once picked, the oils need to be extracted in the right way to be able to provide any type of benefit. In some cases, large quantities of plant yield very little oil. It is for this reason that not all essential oils are as easy to procure.

Some oils, such as cinnamon, clove, orange and ginger are easily available and can be found at reasonable prices. In the case of oils such as jasmine and sandalwood, however, the complicated extraction process means that these oils may be harder to source than others, and may be significantly more expensive to buy.

The scope and reach of aromatherapy in the modern world, however, have made it possible for essential oils to be accessible now more than ever. Today, you can easily find most essential oils readily available at your local health supply stores, or even at online retail websites that provide home delivery.

Chapter 2: The Chemistry behind Aromatherapy

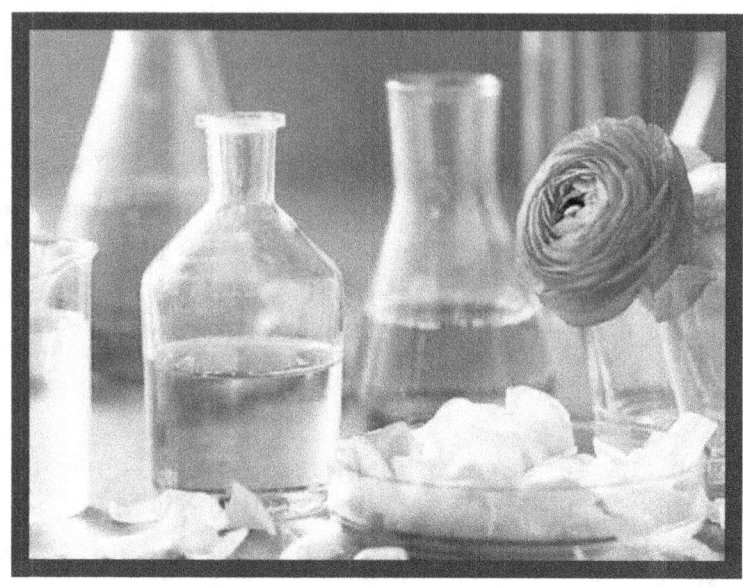

Before our foray into the world of essential oils and Aromatherapy, it's important that you have an understanding of the chemistry behind this science.

Essential oils have distinguishing characteristics that give them different properties, whether they are antiseptic, analgesic, anti-inflammatory, or otherwise. Each of these properties is determined by the chemical nature of that essential oil. To know how to derive the maximum potential from each essential oil, it helps to know the different chemical categories that essential oils are placed in.

Broadly, essential oils are divided into two families based on their chemical structure: Terpene Hydrocarbons and Oxygenated Compounds. Every essential oil is composed of some proportion of Hydrogen, Oxygen and Carbon molecules, which then combine in one of numerous ways to fit into one of the two families. It is important to note, however, that every essential oil may be slotted into more than one of the many categories, based on the properties they exhibit, and their chemical structure.

Let's take a look at the characteristics that each of these families imparts to the essential oils.

Terpene Hydrocarbons

Terpenes are compounds that are a vital part of the chemical structure of an essential oil. It is these compounds that give most oils their antiseptic, antiviral and anti-inflammatory properties. Terpenes are also responsible for de-coagulating blood vessels, as well as restoring tone and structure to muscles and connective tissue.

The following two types are most commonly seen Terpene groups in essential oils:

Monoterpene Hydrocarbons

Monoterpene hydrocarbons are among the most commonly found compounds in essential oils. The main feature of a Monoterpene hydrocarbon is to limit the collection of toxins in your cells. Through this activity, they also help restore the balance of the cellular structure in your body. Monoterpene also act as enhancers, bringing up the potency of other compounds in the essential oil.

These chemical compounds are highly reactive to air and heat, which means that Monoterpene essential oils will have to be stored in airtight, cool conditions. Essential oils with a high level of Monoterpene hydrocarbons include citrus oils such as lemon, orange, and grapefruit, along with others like balsamic fir.

Sesquiterpene Hydrocarbons

Sesquiterpene hydrocarbons are those compounds that provide the anti-inflammatory and antiseptic characteristic to your essential oil. Found in nearly every essential oil, these compounds work by omitting any adverse information from your cellular structure and restoring its original nature.

Sesquiterpene hydrocarbons are also more viscous in nature than their Monoterpene counterparts. This means that they have a thicker texture and are less reactive than Monoterpene. This thicker texture also makes Sesquiterpene essential oils easy to combine with more reactive oils for potent results.

Oils with Sesquiterpene hydrocarbons have found to have a calming, and balancing effect on the mind and emotions as well. Essential oils with high levels of Sesquiterpene include sandalwood, cedarwood, chamomile, rose and myrrh. Oxygenated Compounds

Alcohols

It is the alcohol group of compounds that imparts the energizing or uplifting characteristic to your essential oil. Highly favored in aromatherapy, oils with alcohol compounds are known to have antiviral, antiseptic, and antibacterial properties. The alcohol group also provides a stimulating as well as hypnotic effect to the body, without any side effects or allergic reactions.

Most alcohol-group essential oils can be recognized by their subtle, soft, and often earthy scents. Common examples include geranium, juniper, lavender, tea tree, rose, ginger, vetiver and patchouli.

Aldehydes

Aldehydes are the group that s anti fungal, anti-inflammatory and disinfectant qualities to their essential oils. When used in aromatherapy, oils with Aldehydes can have adaptogenic properties of being calming yet energizing at once.

The use of Aldehydes in aromatherapy requires care and attention to proportions. While extremely beneficial in cures for ailments, they need to be used in highly diluted forms. Potent in small doses, exposure to high amounts of pure Aldehydes may cause allergic skin reactions.

Aldehydes are highly reactive to air and heat. The slightest contact with oxygen or even mildly warm temperatures will bring about a chemical reaction in Aldehydes-group essential oils. Lemongrass, eucalyptus, citronella and melissa are some of the essential oils that belong to the Aldehydes group.

Coumarins and Lactones

Coumarins are the compounds that provide the anticoagulant and sedative properties to their essential oils. Since this compound also imparts its oils with the ability to secret mucus better, Coumarins are highly effective in the treatment of chest-related ailments such as bronchitis.

A sub-type of Coumarins, however, known as furocoumarin, has a highly phototoxic nature. This means that essential oils with furocoumarin compounds become highly reactive and toxic when exposed to long periods of light.

Another group of compounds that is useful in treating chest ailments, yet is phototoxic in nature is a group called Lactones. Lactones also possess anti-inflammatory properties, but can be irritating to the skin upon excessive exposure to light.

Lactones and Coumarins, therefore, need to be used in controlled quantities for short periods of time, and stored away from light. Essential oils that are Coumarins compounds include bergamot, tonka bean, vanilla grass, and sweet grass. Essential oils that contain lactones include jasmine.

Esters

Esters are one of the most cherished among the essential oil compound groups. It is the esters that provide the antispasmodic and relaxing effect to the nervous system and the body. These compounds are formed due to the reactions of alcohols with acids, giving them their calming and sedative properties. The alcohol contribution to the ester group also gives these compounds strongly fragrant characteristics.

Additionally, some ester-group essential oils are have high anti microbial qualities, making them essential in many home treatments. But the feature that makes esters the among the most values essential oil groups is their gentle nature. These compounds mix well with others without bringing about any adverse reactions in the skin. Essential oils with ester compounds include lavender, geranium, bergamot and clary sage.

Ketones

Ketones are those chemical compounds that give their essential oils the ability to enable tissue regeneration and secretion of mucus. These properties are what help your cells and tissue recover faster from injuries and wounds. In addition, treatment with ketones can also help lighten scarring and spots on the skin.

Ketones are a group in the essential oil family tree that need to handled with extreme care. While these oils are highly effective in treatment, they can also be highly toxic. An example of this toxicity is found in the compound Thujone. Found in thuja, which is used in creams to remove stretch marks, excessive exposure to Thujone is known to cause birth defects when used by women.

However, when used in the right amounts and in moderation, kenotic oils have restorative and therapeutic properties that are highly valued. Essential oils with ketone structures include hyssop, rosemary, thuja, wormwood and eucalyptus.

Phenols

Phenols are an important group in the essential oil family tree. These compounds are responsible for a strong fragrance in those oils that belong to the phenol family. Phenol-structured oils are known to have high disinfectant and antiseptic properties. In addition, these oils can also be highly stimulating when used in the correct doses.

The distinguishing feature of phenols is the high number of oxygen molecules they contain. While this makes them effective in improving blood circulation in the body, they also can cause severe reactions when exposed to the skin for too long.

Internally, lengthy periods of treatment with phenolic oils may lead to a toxic buildup, forcing liver damage in the long run.

When used in treatments for a short period in the right amounts, however, phenolic oils can help strengthen and simulate your body and mind, while providing an antiseptic barrier. Essential oils with phenolic properties include cinnamon, clove, wintergreen, thyme and tea tree, among others.

Chapter 3: Embracing the Essential Oils

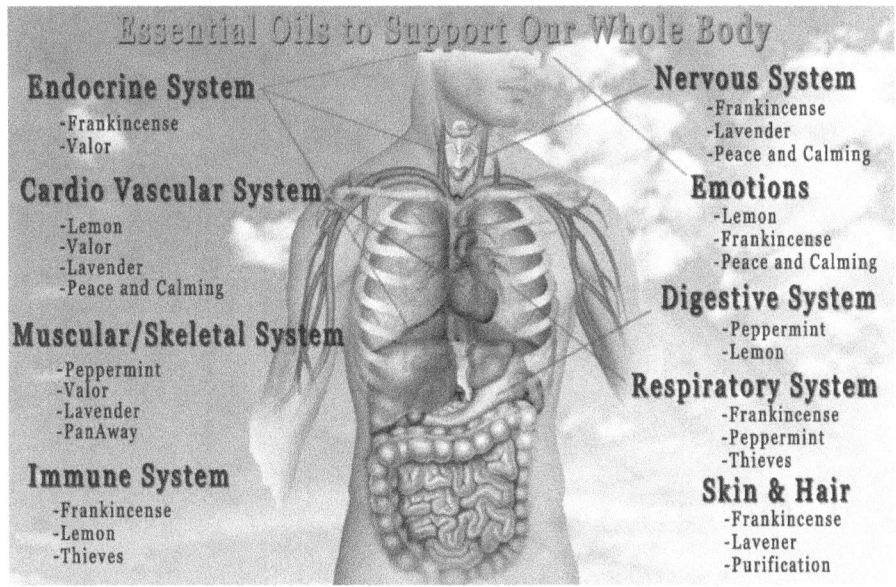

Essential Oils to Support Our Whole Body

Endocrine System
-Frankincense
-Valor

Cardio Vascular System
-Lemon
-Valor
-Lavender
-Peace and Calming

Muscular/Skeletal System
-Peppermint
-Valor
-Lavender
-PanAway

Immune System
-Frankincense
-Lemon
-Thieves

Nervous System
-Frankincense
-Lavender
-Peace and Calming

Emotions
-Lemon
-Frankincense
-Peace and Calming

Digestive System
-Peppermint
-Lemon

Respiratory System
-Frankincense
-Peppermint
-Thieves

Skin & Hair
-Frankincense
-Lavener
-Purification

No matter how much I hype up the essential oils to you, it still falls short of the praise they truly deserve. This group of 300 or so oils, all exhibit a varying range of properties that help treat a host of ailments, both physical and mental. Just some of these powerful properties displayed by essential oils include ones such as:

- Antibacterial

- Antifungal

- Antiviral

- Antiseptic

- Anti-inflammatory

- Antineuralgic

- Antispasmodic

- Antirheumatic

- Antivenemous

- Antitoxic

- Antidepressant

- Sedative

- Nervine

- Analgesic

- Hypotensol

- Hypertensol

- Digestive

- Expectorating

- Deodorizing

- Granulation-stimulating

- Circulation-stimulation

- Diuretic

With properties such as these, is it any wonder that these oils are being turned to for the solution in the field of common ailments and cosmetics. Other industries, such as the culinary and perfumery industries have also switched to these natural sources to add potency to their creations. Through this chapter, you will understand how better to channel the power and potency of these oils into your home. From the essential lists of oils, to information on how to extract them, along with safety guidelines for you, this chapter will broaden your understanding of aromatherapy.

Procuring your Essential and Carrier Oils

When you decide to use the power of essential oils to cure everyday ailments, don't do things halfheartedly. Pay attention to all aspects of the oil so that your blends will be as potent as possible. From the properties of the oil, to the means of extraction, to the pricing itself, every aspect contributes towards finding the right type of essential oils for you.

The first factor to keep in mind when choosing your essential oil, is the purpose of the oil itself. There are twenty different properties exhibited by essential oils, from anti-inflammatory, to antibacterial, to analgesic, antispasmodic, digestive and even deodorizing. When you choose an essential oil, ensure that it has the properties that you need for your ailment. You cannot expect an anti-inflammatory essential oil such as lavender to help with your digestive problems; similarly, aniseed will have little effect as an antidepressant.

Some companies may even try to sell you "combination oils" that smell like one essential oil, but have different effects. For example, carnation is a highly prized essential oil, but is expensive to extract. Therefore, manufacturers will combine the oils of black pepper and ylang ylang, which mimic the scent of carnation, and market it as carnation oil. Steer clear of these combined oils, and buy only pure extracts.

Once you know what essential oils you require ensure that you seek out the purest form of the oil. The purest oils are those that have been extracted from one of the five basic methods: Steam distillation, Enfleurage, Expression, Maceration and Solvent Extraction. These methods have been devised to procure the oil without damaging its essence.

You may find many copies that are marketed as essential oils, but are actually synthetically manufactured in laboratories to replicate the effects of the natural oils. Steer clear of these doppelgangers, as they may do you more harm than benefit.

Another important factor to remember when picking your essential oils is to find a company that does not dilute your oil with carrier oils, unless absolutely necessary. Many companies may try to sell highly diluted versions, while marketing them as concentrates; steer clear of these companies.

An easy way to test if your essential oil has been diluted at the time of packaging is to place a drop of the oil on blotting paper. If the oil leaves a stain behind, that's the carrier oil showing through. Essential oils on their own should only impart the fragrance of the oil, without leaving any stain behind. The only exception to this rule is vetiver, due to its viscous nature.

Perhaps the easiest way to spot a pure essential from a cheap copy, however, is the price of the oil. Since oils have distinct characteristics and methods of extraction, they will not be uniformly priced if they are extracted naturally. When manufactured in a laboratory, these oils are cheap to produce and can be sold for the same price. Your carnation oil should not cost the same as tea tree, just as your jasmine and sandalwood oils will be much costlier than your rosemary or thyme oil.

As you progress through the pages of this book, you will learn more about the extraction processes and uses of the essential oils, which will help you make smarter and well-informed choices for your aromatherapy kit.

Chapter 4: The A-Z of Essential Oils

Essential One-Stop Aromatherapy Chart - Essential Oils

NAME	TYPE	DERIVED FROM	PLACES OF ORIGIN	POWER OF OIL	USE IN THERAPY
Aniseed	herb	seed	India, Indonesia, South America	digestive	cough, bronchitis, indigestion
Bay	tree	leaves	West Indies, South America	antiviral	cold, flu, sprains, insomnia
Bergamot	tree	peel	Morocco, Italy	antidepressant	cough, sores, fever, acne, wounds, tension
Chamomile	herb	leaves/flower	England, France, Hungary, Bulgaria	anti-inflammatory	inflammation, acne, eczema, psoriasis, menstrual issues, dermatitis, migraine, burns
Cinnamon	tree	leaves/twigs	India, Sri Lanka	antiviral	rheumatism, cold, cough, viral infection
Clary Sage	herb	flower	France, Spain	sedative	sore throat, muscular pain, depression

Clove	tree	flower	Philippines, West Indies	analgesic, antiseptic	flatulence, nausea, rheumatism, arthritis, bronchitis, diarrhea, infections, toothache
Eucalyptus	tree	leaves/twigs	China, Australia, Brazil, Spain	anti-inflammatory, antiseptic	cough, sore throat, bronchitis, ulcers, sores, sinusitis, rheumatism, skin infections
Frankincense	tree	bark	China, Somalia, Ethiopia	antiviral, relaxant	wounds, sore throat, colds, fever, bronchitis, laryngitis, stress, tension
Geranium	plant	leaves/stalks/flower	Egypt, China, France, Morocco	antineuralgic	menstrual issues, diarrhea, diabetes, depression, circulatory issues, bleeding, sore throat, kidney

Ginger	plant	root	India, China, Japan, west Africa	digestive	rheumatism, nausea, cold, diarrhea, muscular pains, digestive issues
Grapefruit	tree	fruit rind	United States, Israel	tonic	kidney and liver disorders, migraine, obesity, depression
Hyssop	herb	flower	Brazil, Palestine, south Europe	tonic	rheumatism, arthritis, respiratory issues, cold, cough, sore throat, blood pressure, nervous and circulatory disorders
Jasmine	bush	flower	Egypt, China, France, Algeria, Morocco	relaxant	menstrual issues, laryngitis, lethargy, depression, anxiety
Lavender	plant	flower	France, England	anti-inflammatory, antiviral	rheumatism, arthritis, boils, cuts, wounds, burns, fainting, headaches, nausea, flu, insomnia, bacterial infections, sores, acne, ulcers

Lemon	tree	fruit rind	Israel, Brazil, United States, Argentina	astringent, tonic	sore throat, blood pressure, nervous and digestive disorders, gallstones, anxiety
Lemongrass	grass	plant	Sri Lanka, central Africa, Brazil	tonic, antiseptic, insect repellent	infections, sore throat, respiratory issues, headaches, fever
Lime	tree	fruit rind	Italy, West Indies, Mexico, Brazil	astringent, tonic	fever, rheumatism, headaches, anxiety
Myrrh	tree	bark/resin	Ethiopia, north Africa, Somalia	antibacterial	bacterial and fungal infections, bronchitis, diarrhea
Neroli (Orange Blossom)	tree	flower	Egypt, Italy, France, Morocco, Tunisia	cardiac tonic	depression, hysteria, anxiety, nervous disorders, menopause, dermatitis
Orange	tree	fruit rind	United States, France, Brazil, Spain, India	sedative, antiseptic, tonic	depression, anxiety, nervous conditions, constipation, muscular pains

Oregano	herb	leaves/flower	Egypt, north Africa, parts of Europe, Asia	digestive	rheumatism, bronchitis, muscular pains, respiratory and digestive disorders
Patchouli	plant	leaves	China, Indonesia, Japan	diuretic, antiseptic, insecticide	acne, eczema, dandruff, fungal infections
Peppermint	herb	whole plant	United States, China, parts of Europe	stimulant	indigestion, nausea, flatulence, headaches, migraine, arthritis, liver disorders
Rose	bush	flower	Bulgaria, Morocco	antiseptic, sedative, general tonic	menstrual issues, menopause, circulatory disorders, depression, stress, tension
Rosemary	herb	leaves	Spain, Japan, France	nerve stimulant, cardiac tonic, analgesic, liver decongestant	rheumatism, obesity, dandruff, headaches, muscular pains, sprains, gout, fatigue, spinal injuries, hair fall, skin infections

Sage					
	herb	leaves/flower	China, Mediterranean region	astringent	sores, bronchitis, catarrh, arthritis, rheumatism, fibrositis, sprains
Sandalwood					
	tree	bark	India, Indonesia	sedative antifungal, antibacterial	catarrh, menstrual issues, cystitis, acne, skin infections
Spearmint					
	herb	leaves/flower	United Stated, Russia, Mediterranean region, parts of Europe	digestive	flatulence, nausea, colic, indigestion, intestinal cramps, fever
Tea Tree					
	tree	leaves/twigs	Australia	anti-inflammatory, antibacterial, antifungal, antiviral	cold sores, burns, colds, bacterial and viral infections, warts, acne, shock, hysteria
Thyme					
	herb	flower	Egypt, Mediterranean region	stimulant, general tonic	rheumatism, lethargy, bacterial and urinary sores, wounds
Ylang-ylang					
	tree	flower	Indonesia, Philippines, Comoro Islands	sedative, general tonic	high blood pressure, anxiety, depression

Carrier Oils

Aromatherapy is at its most effective when the essential oils you use are in their purest state. This pure state of the plant material's essence is also highly concentrated - most essential oils are deemed unsafe for use in their raw state. To prepare them for the body, you dilute the oil with a base that will help spread the oil's properties evenly without lessening its potency. The perfect base for this purpose is provided by carrier oils.

Carrier oils or base oils (named for their function), are nothing but pure oils derived from sources in nature, such as nuts, seeds and vegetables, that contain a fatty base. These oils on their won are of high nutritious value. Most of them contain a host of vitamins, such as A, D and E that help maintain excellent skin, nail and hair health. They also contain essential minerals such as calcium, phosphorus, iron, manganese etc, along with healthy fats such as Omega-3 and Omega-6. All these nutrients combine to make carrier oils excellent tools to blend your essential oils with.

In addition, carrier oils generally have a more viscous and thicker texture than the light essential oils. This makes it easy for the essential oil to reach large areas of skin with the same tiny amount and potency. Carrier oils are also less volatile than essential oils, which means that they do not evaporate as easily when in contact with air or heat. Due to this characteristic, they are excellent tools to make your essential oils last longer.

The best ways means of extracting your carrier oils is either through the methods of maceration or cold pressing. Sources for carrier oils are also generally higher-yielding than essential oil sources. This means that you will get more oil from five pounds of olive than you would from five pounds of lavender. It is, however, cheaper and far more convenient to purchase your carrier oils from your local health stores.

When you purchase your carrier oils, ensure that they are extracted through natural means, and not manufactured through synthetic means. Common carrier oils such as olive, coconut and vegetable oil are also used for culinary means. These cooking oils may not have been extracted through a natural source, and will be ineffective in aromatherapy. Try and source your oils from a reputed health store in your area or even online.

Nearly all carrier oils will keep for a long time if stored in a cool and dry area. Since these oils are thicker in texture, you may find that some carrier oils develop a cloudy appearance and firmer texture at low temperatures. This is nothing to worry about; the oils retain their clear, liquid state when the temperature is warmer. The following are a list of the most commonly available carrier oils, with their benefits as well as uses.

Essential One-Stop Aromatherapy Chart - Carrier Oils

NAME	DERIVED FROM	COLOR	USAGE IN BLENDS	RICH IN	USE IN THERAPY
Sweet Almond	kernel	pale yellow	used undiluted	vitamins, minerals, proteins, glucosides	dermal itching, dryness, soreness, inflammation, all skin types
Apricot Kernel	kernel	pale yellow	used undiluted	vitamins, minerals	dermal sensitivity, dryness, inflammation, aging
Avocado	fruit	dark green	10% dilution	vitamins, proteins, fatty acids, lecithin	dermal dehydration, dryness, eczema, all skin types
Borage seed	seed	pale yellow	10% dilution	vitamins, minerals, gamma linolenic acid	aging, psoriasis, eczema, pre-menstrual trauma, menopause, cardiac troubles, cell regeneration, all skin types
Carrot	root	orange	10% dilution	vitamins, minerals, beta-carotene	aging, psoriasis, eczema, itching, dryness, scarring, rejuvenating

Castor	seed	yellow	10% dilution	vitamins, minerals,	dermal itching, dryness, soreness, inflammation, all skin types
Corn	kernel	pale yellow	used undiluted	vitamins, minerals, proteins	all skin types, soothing
Evening Primrose	flower	pale yellow	10% dilution	vitamins, minerals, gamma linolenic acid	aging, psoriasis, eczema, pre-menstrual trauma, menopause, cardiac troubles, cell regeneration, all skin types
Grapeseed	seed	colorless/pale green	used undiluted	vitamins, minerals, proteins	all skin types, soothing
Hazelnut	kernel	yellow	used undiluted	vitamins, minerals, proteins	all skin types, slight astringent
Jojoba	bean	yellow	10% dilution	minerals, proteins, collagen-mimic	psoriasis, eczema, acne, hair fall, penetrating, all skin types,
Olive	fruit	green	10% dilution	vitamins, minerals, proteins	rheumatism, hair care, homemade cosmetics, soothing
Peanut	seed	pale yellow	used undiluted	vitamins, minerals,	all skin types

Safflower	flower	pale yellow	used undiluted	vitamins, minerals, proteins	all skin types
Sesame	seed	dark yellow	used undiluted	vitamins, minerals, proteins, amino acids, lecithin	rheumatism, psoriasis, eczema, arthritis, all skin types
Soya Bean	bean	pale yellow	used undiluted	vitamins, minerals, proteins	all skin types
Sunflower	flower	pale yellow	used undiluted	vitamins, minerals, proteins	all skin types
Wheatgerm	kernel	pale yellow	10% dilution	vitamins, minerals, proteins	all skin types

Chapter 5: Aromatherapy Safety Guide

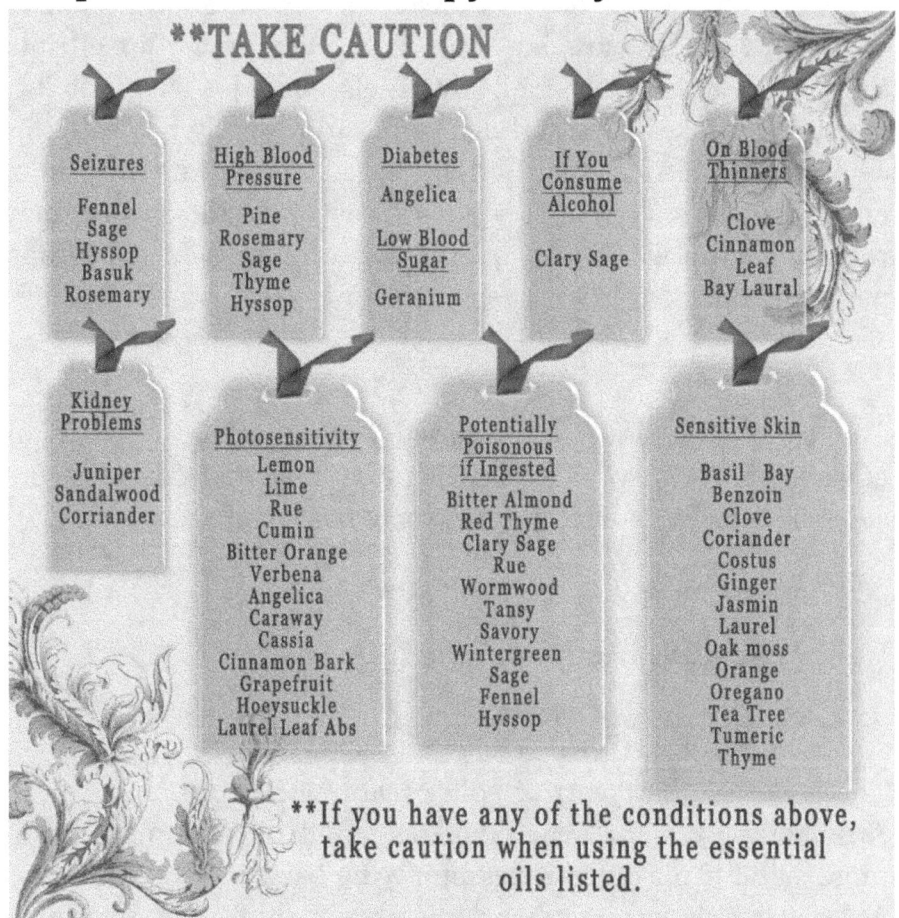

TAKE CAUTION

Seizures	High Blood Pressure	Diabetes	If You Consume Alcohol	On Blood Thinners
Fennel Sage Hyssop Basuk Rosemary	Pine Rosemary Sage Thyme Hyssop	Angelica Low Blood Sugar Geranium	Clary Sage	Clove Cinnamon Leaf Bay Laural

Kidney Problems	Photosensitivity	Potentially Poisonous if Ingested	Sensitive Skin
Juniper Sandalwood Corriander	Lemon Lime Rue Cumin Bitter Orange Verbena Angelica Caraway Cassia Cinnamon Bark Grapefruit Hoeysuckle Laurel Leaf Abs	Bitter Almond Red Thyme Clary Sage Rue Wormwood Tansy Savory Wintergreen Sage Fennel Hyssop	Basil Bay Benzoin Clove Coriander Costus Ginger Jasmin Laurel Oak moss Orange Oregano Tea Tree Tumeric Thyme

If you have any of the conditions above, take caution when using the essential oils listed.

The process of selecting, extracting, blending and then using your essential oils is a carefully cultivated skill. It may take you weeks, even months to familiarize yourself with the vast world of oils, their sources and their benefits. And even then you will have barely scratched the surface of an art that is thousands of years old.

Please don't fret, I do not mean any of these words in a foreboding or discouraging tone! When you ease yourself into the world of Aromatherapy, little else can be as gratifying. However, it takes time and dedication to properly navigate this complex and intricate world. Each oil comes with its own set of quirks and characteristics; some are easy to handle, others may require a little work. Still others may only be safe for certain people and poisonous to others.

To help you avoid any unwanted consequences, mishaps or adverse effects in your experience with essential oils, here are some basic safety guidelines for you to bear in mind:

Never use undiluted essential oils

The reason that carrier oils feature so prominently in Aromatherapy is to help dilute essential oil and make them more suitable for our skin. skipping the basic step of dilution is not a wise choice. You may mistakenly think that undiluted essential oils will be more potent - this is not true. Most essential oils with a phenol or aldehyde component are too concentrated from our skin and may irritate the sensitive layers on contact. A fatty-acid filled base like carrier oils help soften the harshness of the essential oils while delivering the therapeutic effects. Ensure that your essential oils are diluted before use.

Ensure that your sources are natural

As mentioned earlier in this book, essential oils, and their carrier oil counterparts, are most effective when they are pure extracts procured through one of the natural processes. Oils that are synthetically manufactured, or involve the use of any kind of chemicals and processing agents, will most likely irritate your skin. In addition, synthetic oils are also less potent while smelling a little fake. Stick to the handmade or organically sourced essential and carrier oils, and you should have nothing to worry about.

Test the oils for allergies/sensitivities

Since every person has different reactions to the chemical components in essential oils ,it is important to first test the oil on a patch of skin for any allergic reactions or sensitivity. Try a small sample on your skin about 12 hours prior to administering your dose. Any adverse reactions, such as redness, irritation patchiness should appear and disappear instantly. If it persists beyond the 12 hour window, stop using the oil and get medical advice. In case you get some oil into your eyes, clear it away with vegetable oil instead of water.

Reactions to inhaling the fumes of the oils may include nausea, lightheadedness. Disorientation and even a spaced-out sensation. If these do not clear away immediately, take a walk and get some fresh air to help clear your lungs.

Test the oils for phototoxicity and photosensitivity

Ensure that you test your essential oils for phototoxicity before you use them. Oils such as bergamot, along with cold pressed oils such as lemon, lime and grapefruit have varying levels of unwanted reactions when exposed to light or sun lamps. Avoid going outdoors for at least 2 to 4 hours after using any of these oils in aromatherapy and rinse off thoroughly before you step out to avoid adverse reactions.

Never take the oils orally for therapeutic reasons

Do not take in any essential oil internally as a form of therapy or treatment. The only cases in which you may do so are if prescribed by your doctor or an aromatherapist who is extremely professional and licensed in the science of ingesting essential oils for medication. Improper methods of taking in the wrong amount of oil may cause unwanted adverse effects.

Alternate your oil blends

Prolonged use of a particular type of essential oil may not necessarily be a good plan. Most essential oils are highly beneficial when used for a specific amount of time - any longer and they end up causing slight, yet increasing toxic build-ups in your system due to stress on the liver. The best way to avoid this situation is by alternating your essential oil blends regularly. Avoid using the same blend for therapy for over a month; switch your oil and return to it during your next switch-up.

Exercise caution when administering to certain groups of people

While you may be excited to spread your new-found knowledge of aromatherapy around your social circle, know that not all people will have the same reactions to the same groups of oils. Along with watching out for allergic reactions in your patients, also ensure that you have all the necessary information you need beforehand. Avoid recommending your personal blends to elderly people, pregnant women, or those with medical conditions, without consulting their doctors first.

Keep away from the reach of young children

ESSENTIAL OIL CHART FOR CHILDREN

● Avoid use under age 2   ○ Avoid use under age 5   ○ Avoid use under age 5
○ Avoid use under age 10   ● Avoid use on prepubertal children

Basil Berzoin Black Seed Cassia Clove Bud/Leaf/Stern Garlic Ginger Lily
Hyssop Lemon Leaf/Petitgrain Massoia May Chang Melissa/Lemon Balm
Myrtle(honey, aniseed and lemon-Sweet Verbena) Oakmoss Opopanax Oregano
Peru Balsam Saffron Sage (Wild Mountain) Savory Styrax Tea Leaf (Black Tea)
Tea Tree (lemon scented) Treemoss Tuberose Turpentine Verbena (Lemon)

Anise/Aniseed Anise (Star) Fennel (bitter) Fennel (sweet) Myrtle (aniseed)

Cajuput Cardamon Cornmint Galangal (lesser) Ho Leaf/Ravintsara
Laural Leaf/Bay Laurel Marjoram (Spanish) Niaouli Peppermint Rambiazana
Rosemary Sage (Greek/White) Sanna Saro

Eucalyptus

Chaste Tree

Although essential oils are extracted from natural sources and have beneficial properties, they are extremely potent in their undiluted state and should not be ingested in large quantities. For this reason, it is best to store your oils away from the reach of younger and more curious children. Older children should be taught how to differentiate between and handle the oils in your home kit, to prevent any unnecessary incidents.

Know your Dermal Irritants

Some essential oils can be highly irritating to the skin if applied undiluted; they may even be irritating to the skin when diluted with base oils! It is best to try and avoid dermal irritants in your aromatherapy blends as far as possible. If you must use them, ensure that they are balanced with plenty of base oil, along with other anti-inflammatory essential oils. Keep the use of these oils to a minimum to avoid irritating your skin further.

Oils known to be dermal irritants are:

Bay leaf

Cinnamon, bark more than leaf

Clove bud

Citronella

Cumin

Lemongrass

Lemon Verbena

Oregano

Tagetes

Thyme

Safety Guidelines for Pregnant Women

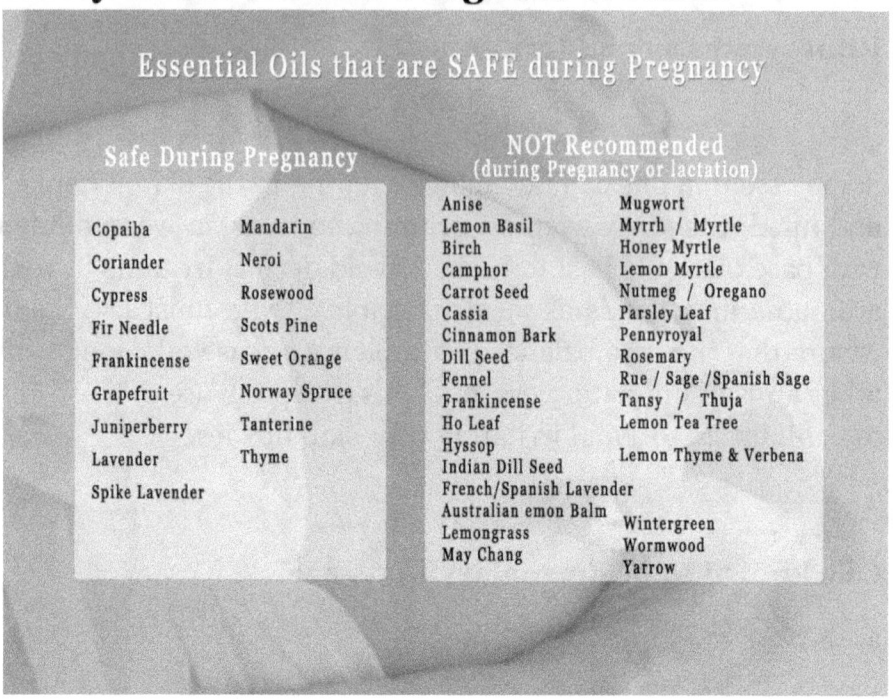

Essential Oils that are SAFE during Pregnancy

Safe During Pregnancy		NOT Recommended (during Pregnancy or lactation)	
Copaiba	Mandarin	Anise	Mugwort
Coriander	Neroi	Lemon Basil	Myrrh / Myrtle
Cypress	Rosewood	Birch	Honey Myrtle
Fir Needle	Scots Pine	Camphor	Lemon Myrtle
Frankincense	Sweet Orange	Carrot Seed	Nutmeg / Oregano
Grapefruit	Norway Spruce	Cassia	Parsley Leaf
Juniperberry	Tanterine	Cinnamon Bark	Pennyroyal
Lavender	Thyme	Dill Seed	Rosemary
Spike Lavender		Fennel	Rue / Sage /Spanish Sage
		Frankincense	Tansy / Thuja
		Ho Leaf	Lemon Tea Tree
		Hyssop	Lemon Thyme & Verbena
		Indian Dill Seed	
		French/Spanish Lavender	
		Australian emon Balm	Wintergreen
		Lemongrass	Wormwood
		May Chang	Yarrow

The use of aromatherapy on pregnant women is considered to be a topic that is still highly debated, with strong arguments for either side of the argument. While many old school of aromatherapy have taught that certain oils, when used during pregnancy result in toxicity and even birth defects, others argue that there are no recorded cases to support this claim.

In many cases, people argue that toxicity to the oils during pregnancy could be the result of large amounts of the oil being used for its benefits. Some oils are known to be good for reducing stretchmarks and carrying related to pregnancy, others are good massage oils. There has been no conclusive evidence determined how safe all the essential oils are for pregnant women, but only a few oils have emerged as pregnancy-friendly.

Here are a list of 15 oils that you should _avoid_ during pregnancy and even during breastfeeding, for your health and your baby's safety:

1. Aniseed

2. Basil

3. Birch

4. Camphor

5. Hyssop

6. Mug wort

7. Parsley seed/leaf

8. Pennyroyal

9. Sage

10. Tansy

11. Tarragon

12. Thuja

13. Wintergreen

14. Wormwood

15. Rosemary

For your safety, it is best to steer clear of all essential oils during the first trimester of pregnancy. During the second and third trimesters, if you must incorporate essential oils in to your massages and other treatments, choose from this restrictive, but gentle list of oils:

1. Rose

2. Neroli

3. Lavender

4. Ylang ylang

5. Chamomile

6. Jasmine

7. Citrus oils like lime, lemon, orange

8. Geranium

9. Sandalwood

10. Spearmint

11. Frankincense

Chapter 6: Creating your Own Aromatherapy Kit

Setting up your aromatherapy kit is probably the most fun part of this organic journey you are taking. The components of your home therapy kit will obviously include all the essential and carrier oils, but the fun factor is added in tracking down these oils.

While there are some carrier oils and essential oils that you can easily extract at home, others may require labor-intensive process to extract and are simply easy to buy from the store instead. Most oils can be easily found at your local health store, or even at your favorite online heath retail store.

When you fill up our kit with the resulting oils, try and add oils that can serve many purposes in a single bottle. Such beneficial oils include lavender, lemon, sandalwood, geranium, tea tree and rose. Start with a few basic oils that address everyday ailments, and then upgrade your kit to include the harder-to-find, rare blend oils.

For your convenience, I have attached a shopping list that lists every oil you might possibly need for your aromatherapy kit. Apart from the oils, you will also find other items such as measuring equipment and blending tools, that help make aromatherapy not only a fun, but also stress-free and relaxing experience.

Essential and Carrier Oils

- Sweet almond oil

- Aniseed oil

- Apricot kernel oil

- Avocado oil

- Bay oil

- Bergamot oil

- Borage seed oil

- Carrot oil

- Castor oil

- Chamomile oil

- Cinnamon oil

- Clary sage oil

- Clove oil

- Corn oil

- Eucalyptus oil

- Evening primrose oil

- Fennel oil

- Frankincense oil
- Geranium oil
- Ginger oil
- Grapeseed oil
- Grapefruit oil
- Hazelnut oil
- Hyssop oil
- Jasmine oil
- Jojoba oil
- Lavender oil
- Lemon oil
- Lemongrass oil
- Lime oil
- Myrrh oil
- Neroli oil
- Olive oil
- Orange oil
- Oregano oil
- Patchouli oil
- Peanut oil

- Peppermint oil

- Rose oil

- Rosemary oil

- Safflower oil

- Sage oil

- Sandalwood oil

- Sesame oil

- Soy Bean oil

- Spearmint oil

- Sunflower oil

- Tea tree oil

- Thyme oil

- Wheatgerm oil

- Ylang ylang oil

Other Aromatherapy kit essentials

- Rolled oats

- Salt

- Liquid castile soap, original or unscented or castile soap flakes

- Measuring spoons

- Glass droppers

- Beakers of various sizes for measurement

- Mixing bowls of various sizes

- Small tubs for hand/foot baths

- Spray dispenser bottles

- Brown glass vials with droppers

- Glass vials with lids

- Safety gloves

- Cooking and body thermometers

- Hot water bottle bag

- Cloth for compresses

- Room diffusers

- Cotton wool

- Stick on labels and markers

Chapter 7: Common Methods of Oil Extraction

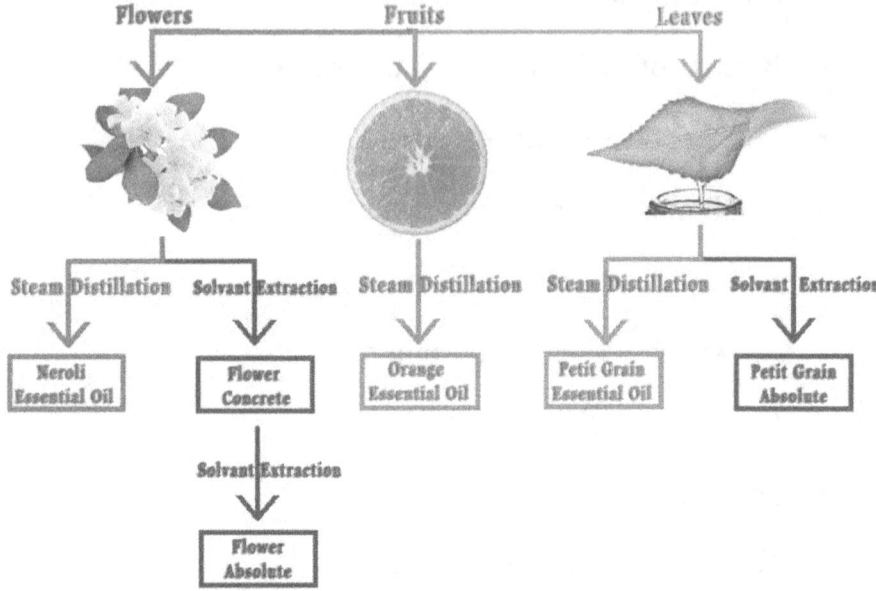

The most intricate and tricky section in the world of aromatherapy is also its most essential one - the process of extraction. When you derive the essence of a natural substance from it, you automatically have several factors that need to be considered. Has the plant material been cultivated the right way? Is it the right time to prepare the plant material for extraction? Can the oils be extracted from the material easily?

And once these questions are answered, there is the actual extraction process. Every plant has a distinct physical structure, and stores its oil deposits in different areas. To get the perfect essential oil, you have to use a means of extraction that can break down the cell walls in the plant to release in the oils from their pockets. This, however, needs to be done without damaging the effects of the plant or altering its chemical structure.

For these purposes, essential oils are mostly extracted on a large-scale basis. The two most common methods used to derive essential oils are steam or water distillation and solvent extraction. Steam distillation and solvent extraction involve placing the plant material either within or above boiling water in a sealed chamber to help extract the essential fumes from the plant. These fumes are collected in a tube and then treated with an ethyl alcohol base to help get the final product.

The problem with these methods, though, is that they need careful monitoring, attention to detail and a specific knowledge of every ingredient involved. And these time-consuming processes may not even give you the amount of oil you require, when undertaken at home.

This doesn't mean that you should try extracting oils at home. There are several methods of extraction that are simple enough to try on easily available plants, like fruit peels, or easily available flowers. Through the following pages, you will learn about three methods - enfleurage, expression and maceration - that help you derive your own oils for aromatherapy from the comfort of your home.

Enfleurage

Enfleurage is an extracted process that was employed in the early days of the perfumery industry. This method was widely practiced in the region of Grasse, France, to extract oils from such flower as jasmine and tuberose.

Oils extracted through these means were highly valued as Enfleurage required vast amounts of work and patience to yield disproportionately low qualities of oil. With the introduction of such modern techniques as solvent extraction, however, Enfleurage became less a less common practice around the world, with Grasse still being one of the last areas known to undertake it.

Enfleurage is one of the gentlest known means of extracting essential oils from plant material. Traditionally, this procedure involved the use of the flower material, along with a readily available form of animal fat or lard. The lard was carefully fit to cover a glass plate - or chassis. The plant material - usually petals from the flower - were then placed and pressed gently onto the lard surface.

The next step required waiting till the oils from the plant material had seeped into the animal fat - this could take days. The plant material was then replaced with a fresh batch and the process was repeated till the fat has absorbed an adequate amount of oil. This oil and wax mixture, called a pomade, was then treated with an ethyl alcohol to separate the fate from the essential oil, resulting in an absolute. This absolute was then diluted and used in therapy and perfumery, while the waxy pomade was used to craft soaps.

Today, this method has been made much simpler and environmentally-conscious by substituting animal fat or lard for a base oil such as olive. Allowing the plant material to float in the base oil for days allows the flower to release oil from its pockets into the container. This infused oil is then treated with ethyl alcohol to separate the absolute from the infusion.

Should you choose to try Enfleurage at home, remember that this process is not labor-intensive, but requires a lot of patience and time. You may find other recipes that tell you infusing the plant material in the base oil yield an essential oil - this is not true. This result is only an infusion - the essence of a plant material is not diluted with other oils and has to be extracted by an agent such as ethyl alcohol. Skipping this alcohol extraction step will give you an oil blend that is not as potent, although it is still therapeutic to an extent.

Oils that can be extracted through this method include flowers such as jasmine, tuberose and lavender.

Maceration

The process of Maceration is that combines the best of Enfleurage with a tweak in the Solvent Extraction method. As with the former, macerating a plant for its essential oil involves soaking the plant material in a carrier oil and then waiting as the oils seep from the plant into the container. The component that distinguishes these two processes is the addition of heat in maceration.

Enfleurage, as we have seen, is used to extract oils from those plant materials that are too volatile or reactive with factors such as heat. When the plant material has a tougher cell membrane that can resist basic reactions, we need to rupture the membrane in order to coax the oil out. A heated base oil is the best means to achieve this without damaging the structure or potency of the essential oil itself.

Like Enfleurage, maceration is a relatively simple extraction procedure to perform at home. Depending on which part of the plant contains the oil, you can use either the whole plant material or the required parts without much preparation. Pay attention to this step as some parts of the plant may contain toxic components not suitable for the human skin.

Another factor to bear in mind during the maceration process is the recommended heat for the base oil. Essential oil can be extracted from different parts of the plant - the stalks, leaves and even roots. Furthermore, the cell membranes of different plants have varied levels of resistance to heat, pressure, light and other variables. Some plants may seep out their oils at relatively low temperatures, while others may need to be soaked in boiling or highly heating oil. Monitor the heating point of your base oils and you should have no problem getting a potent extract.

Oils that can be extracted through the maceration process include plant material such as calendula, carrot, St.John's wort, seaweed, marigold, galangal and horse chestnut.

Expression

The final of the traditional five methods of extracting essential oils is perhaps one off the easiest to perform. Expression, or cold pressing as it commonly known, is the process by which the oil is extracted for the oil-rich rinds of pant material, mostly fruits. Cold pressing is also considered a great way to extract oils from other sources such as nuts and seeds.

Do not be fooled by the appearance of the word "cold" in cold pressing - this is not a heat-free process. While cold pressing will require you to use some measure of heat to help coax the essential oil out from its cell pockets, this heat is relatively low when compared to the other processes of extraction.

When we say cold pressing, we simply mean that the heat applied to the plant material falls between 80 and 120 degrees Fahrenheit - in order to soften up the fleshy oil deposits in the material. The rind, nut or seed is then allowed to set to a cooler temperature before the "pressing" part of the process is undertaken to procure the now loosened oil. The resulting oil may contain some bits from the plant, such as tiny rind pieces, shell fragments or small twigs and seeds. These can easily be filtered away for a clear and pure oil.

The highlight of the cold pressing method is this application of a low heating temperature, as it helps keeps the chemical composition and integrity of the oil intact. The oils extracted through this procedure will often retain their aroma, as well as their color and potency.

Since low levels of heat are required to extract oils through cold pressing, ensure that you pay attention to the temperature on your heating devices, as well as the cooling time required. Along with the quality of plant material used, this attention to heat will affect the quality of your essential oil.

As many manufacturers practice during large-scale expression methods, you can press the same plant material more than once to extract oil until all the oil has seeped out of the cell pockets. Once the first extraction is performed, you simply reheat the plant materials and follow the procedure again till your plant yields no more oil.

This repeated extraction results in oil that may be less potent with each pressing - leading to grades such as "first-pressed", "second-pressed" and so on. If you are purchasing oils extracted through cold processing, try acquiring first-pressed essential oils for the best therapeutic effects.

Oils that can be extracted through the cold pressing methods include citrus plant material such as orange, lime, lemon, grapefruit and bergamot, along with base oils from nuts and seeds like safflower, peanut, flaxseed, pumpkin, sesame, almond and olive.

Chapter 8: Blending your Essential Oils

Once you have assembled your set of oils, both base and carrier, you're ready to make your foray into the next chapter in aromatherapy - the process of blending your oils. We already know that essential oils are generally diluted with base oils to help make them more suitable for our skin. This also helps impart the beneficial properties of the carrier oil. If a mildly diluted form of essential oil with a base can yield a more potent result, imagine the power-packed results that blended essential oils can achieve!

Of course, just like aromatherapy itself, the process of blending is either an inherent gift, or a carefully crafted and cultivated skill. To master blending your essential oils, it is important that you familiarize yourself with the characteristics of the oils themselves. There is enough information available on potent blends that work, so you don't have to succumb to the trial-and-error method. However, once you get the hang of blending oils that complement and enhance their properties, you unlock a limitless treasure trove of cures for daily ailments and health care.

Here are a few important concepts that will help you understand the unique world of essential oil blending better:

Synergy

It is common knowledge that two or more components, when combined effectively, can have greater power than an individual force. This same rule applies in the world of aromatherapy as well. When two or more essential oils with complementary properties, are blended in the right way, we achieve what is called synergy. This state of harmony allows your resulting oil blend to be more potent and therapeutic without increasing the dose of administering

Moreover, the resulting oil blend that you achieve now has its own distinctive properties and characteristics, which help broaden its reach of therapy. Since the purpose of synergy to procure an oil that is of superior quality, you will naturally have to be careful with the oils that you choose to blend.

Important factors to bear in mind are the viscosity and the volatility levels of your essential oils. To achieve synergy, you should find oils that have similar benefits and properties that balance each other out.

As we know, lighter essential oils are more volatile and less viscous in nature. This means that they are thinner in texture while being more aromatic. The heavier oils, on the other hand, are more viscous and less volatile. Therefore, by finding oils that have similar properties while balancing out the volatility and viscosity, you will achieve synergy. An example of a superior blend with synergy is a lavender chamomile blend. While both are antiinflammatory in nature, the lighter chamomile is made more effective and longer-lasting when blended in the right proportion with the heavier lavender.

Adaptogens

Essential oils are classified into groups based on many factors - their chemical composition, volatility, viscosity, phototoxicity, etc. Some oils are antibacterial in nature, others are analgesic. Some oils may have stimulating effects while others may have calming properties. Yet, you may find that some essential oils listed as having opposite effects. Oils that display these multifaceted properties are called adaptogens.

Oils with adaptogenic properties are those that have a balancing effect on your system.These oils are used in the treatment and therapy of areas in your body such as the nervous system, the circulatory system and the endocrine system, to name a few. When you use an adaptogen to treat an ailment, the oil works by neutralizing the ailing effect in your body and bringing your system back to a state of homeostatic balance.

There are a number of essential oils with these unique properties. Hyssop is a popular adaptogen, as it helps to balance out either high or low blood pressure. Peppermint is also famed in the world of aromatherapy for having the dual effects of being both stimulating as well as relaxing. Lemon oil, as well, is a known adaptogen affecting your autonomic nervous system - it can work either as a tonic or as a sedative, based on your need.

Ginseng and mint are essential oils that exhibit their own unique adaptogenic properties.

Chemotypes

We have discussed how variables such as soil, climate, altitude and manner of extraction can affect the resulting essential oil. We also know that plant material may have more than one area to store their oils, which may require many methods of extraction. This may lead to the production of different types of oils from the same plant. When the chemical structure is changed due to any of these factors, it also affects the properties of the oil.

While not all variations may be usable, you are likely to get some oils which have therapeutic properties. They may not have the same potency, but may be more effective at curing another set of ailments, or may find use in another area such as cooking or perfume making. Plant material that can provide more than one distinct oil are known as Chemotypes.

One herb that is a known chemotype is the Thymus Officinalis. This single herb is known to procure several types of oils with distinct medicinal and therapeutic properties, all influenced by factors like altitude, climate and soil. Growing the herb at high altitudes, for instance, will give you Thyme Linalol, the only derivative oil from this herb known to help in pediatric ailments.

Chemotypes require perhaps the most amount of attention to variables, as any change in the method of preparation may give you unintended results.

The Order of Blending your Oils

Essential Oil Dilution

Age / Weight	Recommended Dilution (Total Daily Topical Use)	Dilution %	Approx. Number of EO drops per tsp Carrier Oil
Birth to 12 months (6-22 pounds)	0.3% dilution (up to 1.5 drops EO)		
1-5 years (23-44 pounds)	1.5% to 3% dilution (up to 15 drops EO)	0.3%	1 drop EO per 2 tsp.
6-11 years (45-77 pounds)	1.5% to 5% dilution (up to 17 drops EO)		
12-17 years (78-153 pounds)	1.5% to 20% dilution (up to 25 drops EO)	1.5%	2 drops EO per tsp.
18 or older (154+ pounds)	1.5% dilution to NEAT (up to 45 drops EO)	3%	3 drops EO per tsp.
		5%	5 drops EO per tsp.
		10%	10 drops EO per tsp.
		20%	20 drops EO per tsp.
		33%	33 drops EO per tsp.
		50%	50 drops EO per tsp
		NEAT	EO only, no carrier oil

The essential oil blends you achieve are affected not only by the nature of the oils themselves, but also by how you incorporate their natures into your blending procedure. Certain oils need to be poured in before others as they require more mixing time. Others only need to added in the end as they are added to give the blend synergy and balance. Here is a helpful guideline to follow when blending your oils:

1. Personifiers

These are oils that are first added into your essential oil blend. Personifiers are so-called because they provide a defining characteristic that adds uniqueness to your blend. Personifiers will make up about only up to 5 percent of your blend, but can be spotted by their distinct aromas and long lasting effects. Common personifiers are clary sage and clove.

2. Enhancers

Once you have added the personality-providing essential oil to the bowl, it is time to add in the oil that will enhance the presence of the personifier, both in aroma and effect. Enhancers are characterized by their complementary aromas that are sharp, yet blend well with many oils. These genial properties also extend to their uses - enhancers have properties that blend well with a variety of other oils for potent cures.

An enhancer will make up a large amount of your blend - between 50 to 80 percent - and will provide the maximum amount of therapeutic benefit to your ailment. Popular enhancers in essential oil blends include lemon.

3. Equalizers

You now have two elements in your blend that have sharp aromas and dominant qualities that may be too overpowering. To help balance out these effects, you can add in the next layer of oils - the equalizers.

Aptly named, equalizers are the oils that help balance your oil blend out. Characterized by aromas that are more subtle and effects that last a shorter time, equalizers nevertheless help give your oil blend a well-rounded completion, while providing the same therapeutic effects as other oils. Equalizers such as oregano are commonly used in cosmetic and medicinal blends, and make up anywhere between 10 percent to even half of the oil blend.

4. **Modifiers**

And finally, in case you can tweak your blend in any way to help add more balance and achieve a state of synergy, you can go ahead and use the final group of oil, known as modifiers.

Modifiers are subtly scented oils with short-lasting effects; this does not mean that are not potent, however. These oils are potent when used on their own, but have a greater effect as balancing agents in a complex blended oil. Used in small quantities ranging between 5 and 8 percent, you will recognize modifiers such as grapefruit by their subtle hints in the background against sharper notes of oils such as lavender.

Blending Proportions

While choosing oils to blend together for a mix, remember to first dilute them with a base oil to help make this blend more skin-friendly. Along with making them more suitable, the carrier oils will also increase the shelf-life of your oil blends. While the proportion of carrier oils used in each blend will vary based on their individual properties, here is a basic rule of thumb that you can follow:

- 50-60 drops of your essential oils or oil blends for 1 ounce of carrier oil for therapeutic purposes

- 10-13 drops of essential oil/oil blends for 1 ounce carrier oil fro massage purposes

Tools used while blending oils

If you are taking this much care to ensure that you have the best quality ingredients and the right proportion of each oil, ensure that your blending tools do not deteriorate the quality of your oil. The best material to mix and store your essential oils in is glass.

Glass beakers, droppers and vials are the best options for measurement and storage of oils, as glass does not react with the chemicals in the oils. Furthermore, using glass bowls and wooden utensils to blend your oils is the best way to ensure that their properties are left unaltered. Avoid using metal at all costs. Plastic is also best avoided, although hard plastic may be used when there is no glass alternative.

Chapter 9: Methods of Administering Essential Oils

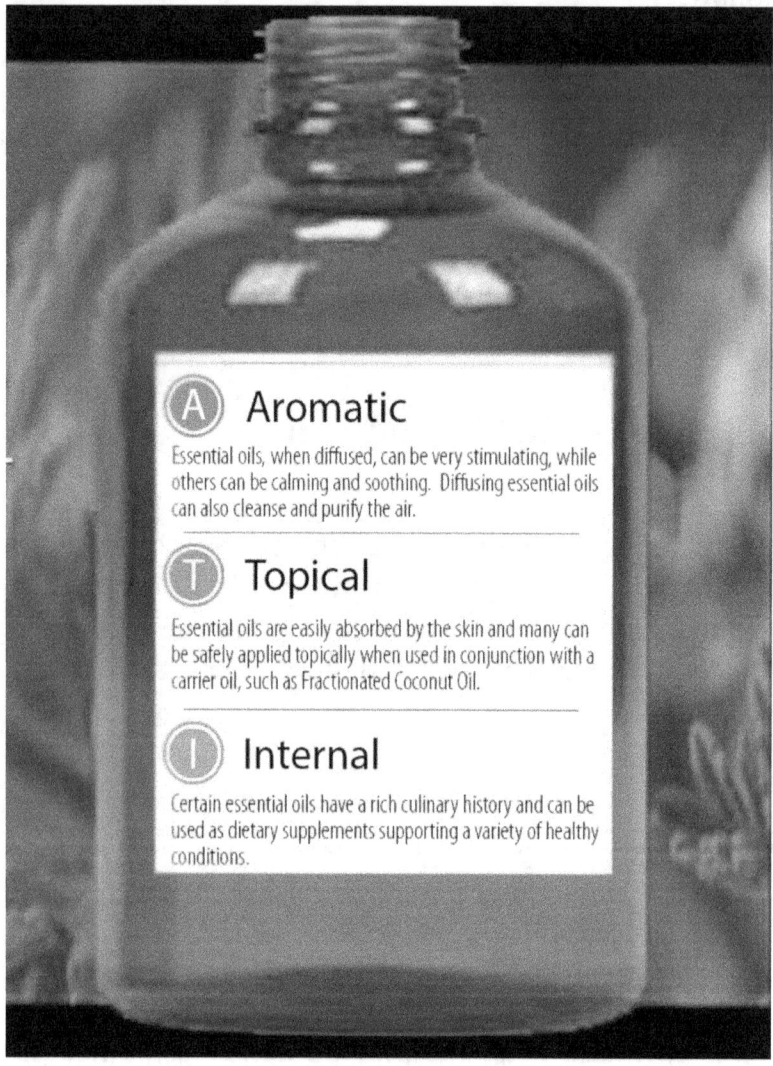

Aromatherapy, as we have already seen, is comprised of a host of essential oils that have various means of cultivation, extraction and blending that influence the resulting therapy they provide. When you do use these oils in your daily life, these multifaceted oils allow for many different methods by which they can be incorporated for therapy or leisure.

The following is a broad categorization of the methods by which you can use your essential oils, based on the means through which they make contact with your body.

Therapy through physical administering

1. Handkerchief/Tissue inhalation

Recommended Dose: 1 drop

How to use: Handkerchief or tissue inhalation is an easy, instant and effective way of administering essential oil therapy to a person, especially in cases that require quick actions, such as breathing difficulties.

1. Apply drop of recommended essential oil or oil blend to clean handkerchief or tissue.

2. Place tissue or handkerchief over nose to cover nasal passages and inhale deeply.

3. Use this mode of therapy as needed.

2. Vapor Inhalation

Recommended Dose: 2-3 drops

How to use: Vapor inhalation is a great way to administer essential oil therapy over a prolonged and relaxed period of time.

1. Fill a bowl large enough to place your face around with hot water.

2. Add the recommended dosage of essential oil to the bowl and mix the contents together well.

3. Place your face over the bowl, about 10 inches away, and cover the back of your head with a large towel. The towel should seal in your face around the bowl on the sides as well.

4. Inhale the steam from the bowl for about 2 minutes.

5. Remove the towel, and breathe normally.

6. Repeat inhalation if necessary.

3. Massage oil

Recommended Dose: up to 5 drops per teaspoon of carrier oil

How to use: Massage oils are the best way to help impart the therapeutic and relaxing properties of many essential oils directly to your skin. The benefits of the oils, combined with the actions of massaging, make this a highly favorable mode of aromatherapy administering.

1. A clean glass bottle is best suited for mixing and storing your massage oils.

2. Add the base oil to the bottle,

3. Follow it up with the recommended essential oil or oil blend.

4. Close the bottle firmly and turn it upside down and back a few times to mix the oils.

5. Then, place the bottle length-wise between your palms and roll it back and forth to ensure the oils have been mixed well.

6. Massage the affected areas as needed.

Therapy through Water

1. Bath

Recommended Dose: up to 8 drops in bath water

How to use: The simplest way to incorporate a session of aromatherapy in your daily routine through water is by soaking in an essential-oil rich bath. For this simply fill up your tub with warm water and add in the oils. Allow around five minutes for the oils to seep in to the water and then immerse yourself and feel the energizing and healing properties of the oils take over.

2. Shower

Recommended Dose: up to 8 drops on scrub pad or loofah

How to use: In case you do not have the time to soak in a daily bath, you can switch up some bath soaks with aromatherapy-rich showers instead.

1. Rinse your body as you normally would.

2. Add the essential oils to the scrub pad or loofah and apply all over body.

3. Scrub oil over skin while under running water to help the oil spread and clean body.

4. Simultaneously, inhale the therapeutic aromas of the oils as you wash them off your body.

5. Rinse off and continue shower as usual.

3. Sauna

Recommended Dose: 1 drop per cup of water

Aromatherapy through sauna is a great way to let the essential oils into your skin, as the oils may enter your body as fumes through inhalation, but lave your body as droplets of sweat through perspiration. This also helps release toxic matter from your system, leading to a healthier skin and body. The best oils to add to your regular sauna sessions include tea tree, pine and eucalyptus, as they are detoxifying, while being relaxing at the same time.

4. Jacuzzi

Recommended Dose: 3 drops per person

If you have an outdoor Jacuzzi, or want to provide a a group Jacuzzi session with a dash of therapeutic goodness, adding essential oils can have not only medicinal, but also emotionally beneficial effects such as calming and relaxing your mind while rejuvenating your senses. Simply add the oil to the water before stepping in and allow about ten minutes for the oils to blend into the water.

5. Hand/foot bath

Recommended Dose: up to 4 drops for hands; up to 6 drops for feet

How to use: many essential oil treatments will not require you to immerse your entire body in water and oil infusions; in these case an area-specific bath, such as a hand or foot bath is ideal.

1. Fill the bowl with warm water.

2. Add the recommended essential oils to the bowl and stir the contents together well.

3. Soak hand or feet in the bowl for about 10 to 20 minutes.

4. Then, rinse thoroughly with plain water and wipe.

Therapy through Air in Room

1. Candles

Recommended Dose: 1-2 drops

How to use: you can easily help diffuse the the properties and aroma of essential oils using candles in your room, without actually making aromatherapy candles.

1. Light a regular wax candle and set it in a candle dish or any other glass dish.

2. Add you essential oil to the melting wax that gathers at the bottom of the dish.

3. Ensure that none of the oil touches the wick of the candle flame. Essential oils are highly flammable.

4. Use a tall candle and add the oil at the bottom.

2. Diffusers

Recommended Dose: 1-6 drops

Diffusers are especially created to help spread the therapeutic fumes of essential oils and are an essential tool in your aromatherapy kit. You will find a variety of diffusers available in different material such as clay, glass and metal. Select a diffuser that has a non-porous plate attached to help you clean it and use more than one oil.

3. Humidifiers

Recommended Dose: 1-9 drops

How to use: Humidifiers provide the perfect means by which to diffuse essential oils into the air of a room without a diffuser.

1. Simply fill the compartment with water and add the essential oil or oil blend to the water compartment of the humidifier.

2. Then run your humidifier as you normally would.

4. Room sprays

Recommended Dose: 4-6 drops per cup water

How to use: room sprays are fairy simple to make and can last up to a month or more when stored in a cool dry place.

1. Find an empty bottle with a spray dispenser.

2. Wash and clean your bottle.

3. Fill it up with one cup of water, followed by 4-6 drops of the recommended essential oil.

4. Close the bottle firmly and shake the contents thoroughly to combine the ingredients.

5. Spray the room as you would regular room spray.

5. Water bowls

Recommended Dose: 1-9 drops per ounce water

How to use: Essential oils can release their aroma and therapeutic properties into the air when allowed to sit in a bowl of hot water. This method works for virtually any essential oil or oil blend and is a cheap alternative if you do not have diffusers at home.

1. Boil an ounce of water in a saucepan on your stove.

2. Add this water to a large glass bowl and allow it to cool for about 2 minutes.

3. Then, add in the essential oil or old blend and gently stir the water to incorporate the oils.

4. Place this bowl in a strategic corner of your room and close all doors and windows.

5. Once the fumes from the oils have blended into the air, you can open the windows again.

6. Wood fires

Recommended Dose: 1 drop oil per wood log

How to use: Essential oils can be relaxing and therapeutic when added to your wood fires. Common oils used in wood fires include cypress, pine, sandalwood and cedarwood.

1. Choose one log from the pile that is to be lit in your fireplace.

2. Add one drop of the oil or oil blend to this log and allow it to soak into the log for at least 30 minutes. You can even add the oil to the log and leave it to soak overnight.

3. Add this log to the fire and light it as usual.

Chapter 10: Essential Oils for Weight Loss

Weight-Loss Essential Oil Blend

Essential Oil	Drops Required
Peppermint	10
Lime	30
Tangerine	45
WIld Orange	45
Lemon	75
Grapefruit	75

Store drops in glass bottle, preferably in a dark cupboard.
Use approximately 7 drops before meals (mix in water or put into a Veggie Capsule) and be sure to drink at "Least" 16 0z of water with the oils.

At some point or the other, each one of us has looked in the mirror and wished we were just a couple of pounds lighter. "Maybe I could have a flatter tummy", you might think. Or you may curse yourself for having an appetite that never seems to be satisfied. The problem with losing those few extra pounds, however, is that it usually requires either physical exercise, or tons of money in the form of expensive treatments.

Here is where aromatherapy comes in handy, yet again. Many weight loss treatments rely on vitamins, minerals and antioxidants that help to curb your appetite, reduce your craving for substances like sugar and fat, and help tone up your body. But why turn to expensive treatments when your aromatherapy kit has every agent you need to help with your battle against those extra pounds?

Through this chapter, you will learn simple remedies that help combat weight loss by attacking the factors that contribute to weight gain. Therefore, you will find a recipe that helps to overcome stress eating or impulse eating. There are ideas to help maintain a full and content feeling after a meal, as well as one recipe that helps to reduce metabolism. You will also find an idea that helps in detoxification and breakdown of fatty substances in your body, along with another one to help keep cravings under control.

Aromatherapy for food cravings

Oils you will need:

- 10 drops cinnamon oil

- 10 drops bergamot oil

- 1 tablespoon coconut oil

Methods of application:

1. Add them to a small mixing bowl and stir to combine them well together.

2. Massage you feet with a few drops of this oil to help curb appetite and keep you feeling full after meals.

3. Alternatively, you can add up to 8 drops of this blend in your bath, Jacuzzi, or even in your room into your diffusers.

Aromatherapy for digestive detoxification

Oils you will need:

- 10 drops peppermint oil

- 5drops lemon oil

- 1 tablespoon almond oil

Methods of application:

1. Add them to a small mixing bowl and stir to combine them well together.

2. Massage you feet with a few drops of this oil.

3. Alternatively, you can add up to 8 drops of this blend in your bath, Jacuzzi, or even in your room into your diffusers.

Aromatherapy for metabolism control

Oils you will need:

- 5 drops cinnamon oil

- 5 drops grapefruit oil

- 2 drops lemon oil

- 2 tablespoons olive oil

Methods of application:

1. Add them to a small mixing bowl and stir to combine them well together.

2. Massage your abdomen and feet with a few drops of this oil to help enhance metabolism and break down food substances easily.

3. Alternatively, you can add up to 8 drops of this blend in your bath, Jacuzzi, or even in your room into your diffusers.

Aromatherapy for overeating and stress eating

Oils you will need:

- 10 drops bergamot oil

- 10 drops sandalwood oil

- 2 tablespoons olive oil

Methods of application:

1. Measure out the required oils.

2. Add them to a small mixing bowl and stir to combine them well together.

3. Massage you feet with a few drops of this oil to help calm your nerves down and curb any behaviors that result from stress and anxiety, such as overeating.

4. Alternatively, you can add up to 8 drops of this blend in your bath, Jacuzzi, or even in your room into your diffusers.

Aromatherapy to help enhance weight loss

Oils you will need:

- 10 drops cinnamon oil

- 10 drops grapefruit oil

- 8 drops ginger oil

- 2 tablespoons apricot kernel oil

Methods of application:

1. Add them to a small mixing bowl and stir to combine them well together.

2. Massage you feet with a few drops of this oil to help keep your appetite levels low, consistent and balanced.

3. Alternatively, you can add up to 8 drops of this blend in your bath, Jacuzzi, or even in your room into your diffusers.

Chapter 11: Aromatherapy for Common Ailments

Aromatherapy for aches and pains

Headache
Oils you will need:

- 2 drops rosemary oil

- 1 drop peppermint oil

- 3 drops lavender oil

- 1 tablespoon carrier oil

Methods of application:

1. Measure out the required oils.

2. Add them to a small mixing bowl and stir to combine them well together.

3. Apply up to two drops of the oil blend to the affected area and massage thoroughly for a few minutes.

Stomach and abdominal ache
Oils you will need:

- 3 drops peppermint oil

- 2 drops clove oil

- 2 drops eucalyptus oil

- 1 tablespoon carrier oil

Methods of application:

1. Measure out the required oils.

2. Add them to a small mixing bowl and stir to combine them well together.

3. Apply up to two drops of the oil blend to the affected area and massage thoroughly for a few minutes.

Aromatherapy for cold, cough and flu

Common cold

Oils you will need:

- 3 drops lemon oil

- 1 drop lemon oil

- 2 thyme oil

- 2 tea tree oil

Methods of application:

1. Measure out the required oils.

2. Add them to a small mixing bowl and stir to combine them well together.

3. Add up to 8 drops of this blend in your bath, and even in your room into your diffusers.

Cough

Oils you will need:

- 1 drop eucalyptus oil

- 1 drop thyme oil

- 3 drops tea tree oil

- 2 drops lavender oil

Methods of application:

1. Pick any of the above mentioned oils most easily available to you, or make a blend with a drop of each oil

2. Drop this oil blend onto a handkerchief or tissue and inhale deeply to help revive person from a dizzy spell.

3. You can also use this blend by adding it to a bowl filled with warm water before inhaling the fumes through the steam inhalation process.

Flu

Oils you will need:

- 5 drops tea tree oil

- 2 drops lavender oil

- 2 drops thyme oil

Methods of application:

1. Measure out the required oils.

2. Add them to a small mixing bowl and stir to combine them well together.

3. Add up to 8 drops of this blend in your bath, and even in your room into your diffusers.

Aromatherapy for ear-related ailments

Ear ache

Oils you will need:

- 3 drops chamomile oil

- 1 drop lavender oil

- 1 drop tea tree oil

- 1 teaspoon carrier oil

Methods of application:

1. Measure out the required oils.

2. Add them to a small mixing bowl and stir to combine them well together.

3. Apply up to two drops of the oil blend to the affected area and massage thoroughly for a few minutes.

Ear infection

Oils you will need:

- 3 drops tea tree oil

- 1 drop thyme oil

- 2 drop lavender oil

Methods of application:

1. Measure out the required oils.

2. Add them to a small mixing bowl and stir to combine them well together.

3. Apply up to two drops of the oil blend to the affected area and massage thoroughly for a few minutes.

Aromatherapy for dental ailments

Toothache

Oils you will need:

- 3 drops chamomile oil

- 1 drop clove oil

- 1 lemon oil

- 1 teaspoon carrier oil

Methods of application:

1. Measure out the required oils.

2. Add them to a small mixing bowl and stir to combine them well together.

3. Apply up to two drops of the oil blend to the affected area and massage thoroughly for a few minutes.

Mouth ulcers

Oils you will need:

- 2 drops peppermint oil

- 4 drops lemon oil

- 2 drops geranium oil

Methods of application:

1. Measure out the required oils.

2. Add them to a small mixing bowl and stir to combine them well together.

3. Apply up to two drops of the oil blend to the affected area and massage thoroughly for a few minutes.

Aromatherapy for emergency first-aid

Boils

Oils you will need:

- 2 drops lavender oil

- 2 drops tea tree oil

- 1 teaspoon carrier oil

- 250 ml warm water

Methods of application:

1. Measure out the required oils.

2. Add them to a wide bowl filled with warm water and stir to combine them well together.

3. Bathe the affected area in this water and oil mix for about five to ten minutes once a day till the area is healed.

Blisters

Oils you will need:

- 1 drop lavender oil

- 1 drop chamomile oil

- 1 teaspoon carrier oil

Methods of application:

1. Measure out the required oils.

2. Add them to a small mixing bowl and stir to combine them well together.

3. Apply up to two drops of the oil blend to the affected area.

Bruises

Oils you will need:

- 2 drops geranium oil

- 2 rose oil

- 1 drop lavender oil

- 1 teaspoon carrier oil

Methods of application:

1. Measure out the required oils.

2. Add them to a wide bowl filled with warm water and stir to combine them well together.

3. Bathe the affected area in this water and oil mix for about five to ten minutes once a day till the area is healed.

Cuts and Wounds

Oils you will need:

- 5 drops lavender oil

- 2 drops tea tree oil

- 2 cups warm water

Methods of application:

1. Measure out the required oils.

2. Add them to a wide bowl filled with warm water and stir to combine them well together.

3. Bathe the affected area in this water and oil mix for about five to ten minutes once a day till the area is healed.

4. You can also use this blend to make a compress and place it on the affected area for about thirty minutes till the wound has healed.

Insect bites and stings

Oils you will need:

- 10 drops lavender oil

- 10 drops eucalyptus oil

- 10 chamomile oil

- 10 drops thyme oil

- 2 tablespoons carrier oil

Methods of application:

1. Measure out the required oils.

2. Add them to a small mixing bowl and stir to combine them well together.

3. Apply up to two drops of the oil blend to the affected area.

Cold sores

Oils you will need:

- 10 drops geranium oil

- 10 drops lavender

- 8 drops lemongrass oil

- 2 tablespoons carrier oil

Methods of application:

1. Measure out the required oils.

2. Add them to a small mixing bowl and stir to combine them well together.

3. Apply up to two drops of the oil blend to the affected area.

Frostbites

Oils you will need:

- 4 drops geranium oil

- 2 drops clove oil

- 1 teaspoon carrier oil

Methods of application:

1. Measure out the required oils.

2. Add them to a small mixing bowl and stir to combine them well together.

3. Apply up to two drops of the oil blend to the affected area.

Aromatherapy for rejuvenating after episodes of fainting

Oils you will need:

- 2 drops chamomile oil

- 1 drop lavender oil

- 1 drop geranium oil

Methods of application:

1. Pick any of the above mentioned oils most easily available to you, or make a blend with a drop of each oil

2. Drop this oil blend onto a handkerchief or tissue and inhale deeply to help revive person from a dizzy spell.

3. You cal also use this blend by adding it to your bath for an extra shot of rejuvenation after a spell of unconsciousness.

Aromatherapy for hiccups and halitosis

Essential oils for Hiccups

Oils you will need:

- 1 drop chamomile oil

- 1 drop lavender oil

- 1 drop lemon oil

Methods of application:

1. Pick any of the above mentioned oils most easily available to you, or make a blend with a drop of each oil

2. Drop this oil blend onto a handkerchief or tissue and inhale deeply till hiccups subside.

Essential oils for Halitosis

Oils you will need:

- 2 drops tea tree oil

- 2 drops peppermint oil

- 2 drops lemon oil

- 2 drops lavender oil

Methods of application:

1. Pick any of the above mentioned oils most easily available to you, or make a blend with a drop of each oil

2. Drop this oil blend onto a handkerchief or tissue and inhale deeply till your mouth is deodorized completely.

3. You can also mix this blend with 1 tablespoon apple cider vinegar to make a quick deodorizing rinse.

Aromatherapy for constipation

Oils you will need:

- 15 drops rosemary oil

- 10 drops lemon oil

- 5 drops peppermint oil

- 2 tablespoons carrier oil of your choice

Methods of application:

1. Measure out the required oils.

2. Add them to a small mixing bowl and stir to combine them well together.

3. Store the resulting blend in a glass bottle with a cover.

4. Use this oil to give your abdominal area a massage when affected by symptoms of constipation to feel relief within hours.

Chapter 12: Aromatherapy for a Youthful and Rejuvenated Body

Essential oils are not just effective in helping to relieve symptoms of ailments or treat disorders and conditions. These set of oils are also beneficial in the world of beauty and general physical care. Packed with all the essential vitamins, minerals and proteins, essential and carrier oils can combine to make blends that address all your skin care, hair care and other daily needs better than chemically- manufactured products.

Through this chapter, you will learn to make your own simple blends for daily facial cleansers and scrubs. You will also learn to concoct your own shampoos for regular wash, dandruff treatment and hair fall eradication. This chapter also addresses oil blends that are safe to use during and after pregnancy, along with giving you a blend to help alleviate menstrual pains.

Aromatherapy blend for anti-aging

Oils you will need:

- 10 drops neroli oil

- 10 drops frankincense oil

- 10 drops evening primrose

- 10 drops fennel oil

- 10 drops lavender oil

- 3 drops lemon oil

- 2 drops rosemary oil

- 2 tablespoons sweet almond oil

Methods of application:

1. Measure out the required oils, both essential and carrier.

2. Add the almond oil to a small mixing bowl or directly into a bottle with a flip-cap.

3. Mix the above mentioned essential oils into this almond oil base by stirring them together, or closing the bottle cap and shaking to blend the oils.

4. Store the resulting blend in a glass bottle with a cover.

5. Use this oil to give your face, arms, legs and neck a daily 5 minute massage to combat all the signs of aging that show on skin.

Aromatherapy for cellulite buildup due to aging

Oils you will need:

- 10 drops grapefruit oil

- 10 drops cinnamon oil

- 5 drops ginger oil

- 3 drops lemon oil

- 2 drops rose oil

- 2 tablespoons sweet almond oil

Methods of application:

1. Measure out the required oils, both essential and carrier.

2. Add the almond oil to a small mixing bowl or directly into a bottle with a flip-cap.

3. Mix the above mentioned essential oils into this almond oil base by stirring them together, or closing the bottle cap and shaking to blend the oils.

4. Store the resulting blend in a glass bottle with a cover.

5. Use this oil to give affected areas a daily 10-15 minute massage to to help tone up the skin and reduce the appearance and buildup of cellulite.

Aromatherapy for youthful skin

Oils you will need:

- 1 tablespoon apricot kernel oil

- 10 drops rose oil

- 8 drops carrot oil

- 10 drops geranium oil

Methods of application:

1. Measure out the required oils, both essential and carrier.

2. Add the apricot kernel oil followed by the carrot oil and stir combine them together.

3. Mix the above oils with rose and geranium oils. Continue to stir to form a fragrant blend.

4. Store the resulting blend in a glass bottle with a cover.

5. Use this oil to give your face, arms, legs and neck a daily 5 minute massage for a youthful complexion.

Aromatherapy for facial care

Facial scrubs

Oils you will need:

-   1 teaspoon ground oats

-   1/4 teaspoon salt

-   1/2 teaspoon apple cider vinegar

-   1 drop basil oil

Methods of application:

1. Measure out the required oils and oats.

2. Add them to a small mixing bowl and stir to combine

them well together.

3. Mix the above oils with salt and apple cider vinegar. Continue to stir to form a coarse-textured paste.

4. Apply to your face and scrub for a minute or two.

5. Rinse thoroughly with lots of water and apply a moisturizer after.

Facial cleansers

Oils you will need:

1. 4 drops sesame oil

2. 4 drops sunflower oil

3. 1 tablespoon wheatgerm oil

Methods of application:

1. Measure out the required oils.

2. Add them to a small mixing bowl and stir to combine them well together.

3. Store the resulting blend in a glass bottle with a cover.

4. Use this oil as a daily face cleanser to clear away pollution-created toxins and make up.

Essential oils for facial wrinkles

Oils you will need:

- 2 drops patchouli oil

- 8 drops rose oil

- 5 drops carrot oil

- 5 drops Borage seed oil

- 5 drops jojoba oil

- 2 tablespoon almond or apricot oil

Methods of application:

1. Measure out the required oils.

2. Add them to a small mixing bowl and stir to combine them well together.

3. Store the resulting blend in a glass bottle with a cover.

4. Use this oil to give your face and other areas affected by signs of aging like wrinkles a daily 5 minute massage.

Aromatherapy for hair care

Oils for Dandruff

Oils you will need:

- 250 ml liquid castile oil

- 10 drops thyme oil

- 18 drops rose oil

- 3 drops sage oil

Methods of application:

1. Get out a glass bottle preferably with a spray dispenser cap.

2. Add all the ingredients to the bottle and cover it firmly.

3. Shake the bottle to blend the ingredients together well.

4. Use this shampoo twice a week for best results.

Oils for hair fall

Oils you will need:

- 250 ml liquid castile oil

- 2 tablespoons almond oil

- 4 drops Borage seed oil

- 2 drops chamomile oil

Methods of application:

1. Get out a glass bottle preferably with a spray dispenser cap.

2. Add all the ingredients to the bottle and cover it firmly.

3. Shake the bottle to blend the ingredients together well.

4. Use this shampoo twice a week for best results.

Oils for normal hair wash

Oils you will need:

- 250 ml liquid castile oil
- 4 drops rose oil
- 2 drops lemon oil
- 4 drops eucalyptus oil

Methods of application:

1. Get out a glass bottle preferably with a spray dispenser cap.
2. Add all the ingredients to the bottle and cover it firmly.
3. Shake the bottle to blend the ingredients together well.
4. Use this shampoo twice a week for best results.

Aromatherapy for pregnant and nursing women

Pregnancy Massage Blend

Oils you will need:

- 10 drops Borage seed oil

- 5 drops carrot oil

- 2 tablespoons almond oil

- 1 tablespoon wheatgerm oil

Methods of application:

1. Measure out the required oils.

2. Add them to a small mixing bowl and stir to combine them well together.

3. Mix the above oils with 2 tablespoons of almond oil followed by the wheatgerm oil. Massage the affected areas two to three times a day with this blend.

Essential oils for pregnancy cramps

Oils you will need:

- 10 drops lavender oil

- 5 drops geranium oil

- 2 drops cypress oil

- 2 tablespoon olive oil

Methods of application:

1. Measure out the required oils.

2. Add them to a small mixing bowl and stir to combine them well together.

3. Mix the above oils with 2 tablespoons of a carrier oil such as olive or vegetable Massage the affected areas two to three times a day with this blend.

Essential oils for postnatal massage

Oils you will need:

- 9 drops frankincense

- 6 drops rose oil

- 2 drops lemon oil

- 2 tablespoons olive or vegetable oil

Methods of application:

1. Measure out the required oils.

2. Add them to a small mixing bowl and stir to combine them well together.

3. Mix the above oils with 2 tablespoons of a carrier oil such as olive or vegetable Massage the affected areas two to three times a day with this blend.

Aromatherapy for menstrual issues

Oils you will need:

- 10 drops bergamot oil

- 10 drops geranium oil

- 9 drops rose oil

- 12 drops clary sage oil

Methods of application:

1. Measure out the required oils.

2. Add them to a small mixing bowl and stir to combine them well together.

3. Add up to 8 drops of this blend in your bath, Jacuzzi, or even in your room into your diffusers.

4. You can also mix the above oils with 2 tablespoon of a carrier oil such as almond, olive or jojoba and massage your abdominal area.

Chapter 13: Aromatherapy for your Mind and Soul

Aromatherapy is so effective in the relieving and treatment of everyday physical ailments, as we have just seen in the previous chapters. These oils also help to nurture and pamper your skin, along with maintaining the beauty of your nails, hair and complexion. Along with these physical benefits, however, essential oils are alps highly therapeutic for your mind.

In your daily routine, incorporate one of these essential oil blends to feel the difference that aromatherapy can make to your mood and emotional state. You will find a blend that help keep your office space sterilized, as well as filled with a productive buzz. You will also find a blend each that helps you rejuvenate first thing in the morning or relax after a long day at work. Finally, you will also discover an oil blend that helps alleviate anxiety and calm you down completely.

Aromatherapy to relieve stress

Essential oil blend 1

Oils you will need:

- 10 drops ginger oil

- 11 drops geranium oil

- 9 drops bergamot oil

Methods of application:

1. Measure out the required oils.

2. Add them to a small mixing bowl and stir to combine them well together.

3. Add up to 8 drops of this blend in your bath, Jacuzzi, or even in your room into your diffusers.

Essential oil blend 2

Oils you will need:

- 15 drops grapeseed oil

- 11 drops rose oil

- 3 drops lavender oil

Methods of application:

1. Measure out the required oils.

2. Add them to a small mixing bowl and stir to combine them well together.

3. Add up to 8 drops of this blend in your bath, Jacuzzi, or even in your room into your diffusers.

Aromatherapy for your office space

Oils you will need:

- 10 drops tea tree oil

- 5 drops lavender oil

- 8 drops rose oil

- 5 drops grapeseed oil

Methods of application:

1. Measure out the required oils.

2. Add them to a small mixing bowl and stir to combine them well together.

3. Store this blend in a small glass bottle and carry to work.

4. Add up to 8 drops of this blend into a humidifier or diffuser for your office space.

5. You can even mix this blend into a bowl of warm water and leave it in a corner of your office or on the desk.

Aromatherapy to overcome anxiety

Oils you will need:

- 10 drops lavender oil

- 10 drops geranium oil

Methods of application:

1. Measure out the required oils.

2. Add them to a small mixing bowl and stir to combine them well together.

3. Add up to 8 drops of this blend in your bath, Jacuzzi, or even in your room into your diffusers.

Aromatherapy for rejuvenation

Oils you will need:

- 10 drops lemon oil

- 15 drops lavender oil

- 5 drops clary sage oil

Methods of application:

1. Measure out the required oils.

2. Add them to a small mixing bowl and stir to combine them well together.

3. Add up to 8 drops of this blend in your bath, Jacuzzi, or even in your room into your diffusers.

Aromatherapy for relaxation

Oils you will need:

- 10 drops sandalwood oil

- 10 drops lavender oil

- 5 drops bergamot oil

- 5 drops rose oil

Methods of application:

1. Measure out the required oils.

2. Add them to a small mixing bowl and stir to combine them well together.

3. Add up to 8 drops of this blend in your bath, Jacuzzi, or even in your room into your diffusers.

Chapter 14: Aromatherapy for your Home and Hearth

Since we have incorporated essential oils and aromatherapy into our daily lives through treating physical and mental ailments, why not spread the goodness of the oils into other areas of the household as well?

We have already learned how essential oils have repellent and antibacterial properties, along with being excellent cleansing agents. Due to these reasons, they make for excellent tools to your home cleaning kit. Through this chapter you will find solutions to help clean stubborn surfaces in your kitchen and bathrooms, as well as find an easy blend to help scrub your dishes more effectively.

You will also find a number of oil blends to help add freshness and the right setting to your living rooms and bedrooms. We haven't forgotten the non-human members of your family! You will also discover essential oil blends for daily care for pets, as well as for your garden.

Aromatherapy for your living room and bedrooms

Light and Stimulating oil blend

Oils you will need:

- 10 drops lemon oil

- 4 drops geranium oil

- 2 drops sandalwood oil

Methods of application:

1. Collect a spray dispenser bottle.

2. Add all the ingredients to this bottle and cover it firmly.

3. Shake the contents and it is ready for use!

Earthy and Relaxing oil blend

Oils you will need:

- 8 drops orange oil

- 3 drops frankincense oil

- 4 drops geranium oil

Methods of application:

1. Collect a spray dispenser bottle.

2. Add all the ingredients to this bottle and cover it firmly.

3. Shake the contents and it is ready for use!

Aromatherapy for your Kitchen

Essential oil blend for kitchen surfaces and counter-tops

Oils you will need:

- 10 drops lemon oil

- 8 drops lavender oil

- 8 drops rosemary oil

- 5 drops eucalyptus oil

- 2 tablespoons white vinegar

- 1/2 cup water

Methods of application:

1. Collect a spray dispenser bottle.

2. Add all the ingredients to this bottle and cover it firmly.

3. Shake the contents and it is ready for use!

Essential oil blend to scrub the dishes

Oils you will need:

- 5 drops lime oil

- 3 drops Borage seeds oil

- 2 drops lavender oil

- 1 drop orange oil

- 1 tablespoon white vinegar

- 1/2 cup water

Methods of application:

1. Add all the ingredients to a clear bottle and cover it firmly.

2. Shake the bottle well to combine the ingredients.

3. Use the blend to scrub and rinse your dishes to give them an antibacterial coating.

Aromatherapy for regular health care for pets

How to use Essential Oils with Pets

- Diffusing – Ensure your animal is able to move away from the diffuser it they do not like it.

- Petting – Take 1 drop of oil in your hands, rub them together until no residue is left on your palm & pet your animal. Avoid the sensitive areas of their face, nose, or the bottoms of their feet.

- Internally – Start with 1 drop in their water or food. You can mix with NingXia Red, coconut oil, honey or red agave.

- Indirect – Place 1 drop in your palm, rub in, and then rub onto something your pet can approach (bedding or the perch of a bird cage).

- Water Misting – Add 4 oz. of water and 1 drop of oil into a glass spray bottle. Shake well & then mist.

- Oil Misting – Mix an oil with a carrier oil in a glass spray bottler & spray your pet. (1:4 ratio)

- Topically – Allow 1 drop of oil to drip right onto the animal

- Raindrop – Similar to the human raindrop technic were you drip oils along the spine from tail to head

Peppermint: beneficial when used with wintergreen and clove essential oils on minor injuries for general aches and pains. Use 1 drop in water when out on a hot day. *Cats must have this oil diluted before use.

Lavender: great for minor injuries. Gentle for cleansing. I add it to a spray bottle (1 part lavender to 2 parts water) and shake, great for keeping mosquitoes off. Peppermint increases healing while decreasing aches and pains. It repels parasites and calms the nervous system as it aids in skin and tissue health.

Thieves (contains rosemary, cinnamon bark, cloves, lemon and eucalyptus) is ideal for treating minor injuries, dental issues, is wonderful for supporting their immune sytstem, great for ticks and safe to use both topically and internally.

Frankincense (cold pressed from the fresh lemon peels) is safe and gentle for smaller pets and even birds. Is is used for wounds, skin and tissue health as well as behaviour issues, fungus, general cleaning and more!

Panaway (wintergreen and clove essential oils) is an all round great blend for minor injures, urinary health, aches and pains, dental work recovery. Use topicaly with a warm compress or on the paws (see chart below). *Always dilute before using on cats.

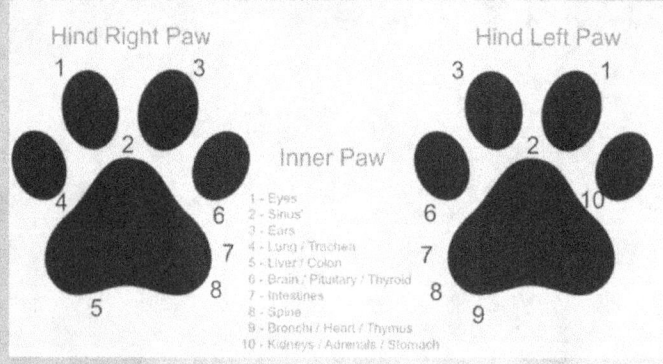

Essential oil blend for bad breath

Oils you will need:

- 1 drop clove oil

- 1 drop lavender oil

- 1 drop myrrh oil

- 1 teaspoon vegetable oil

Methods of application:

1. Measure out a drop of the clove, lavender and myrrh oils.

2. Add these measured oils to a small mixing bowl and follow it up with the vegetable oil.

3. Mix them well to combine them together and then add the blend to your pet's feed.

Essential oil blend for a shiny coat

Oils you will need:

- 1 tablespoon olive oil

- 1 tablespoon wheatgerm oil

- 5 drops carrot oil

- 5 drops evening primrose oil

Methods of application:

1. Measure out five drops each of the carrot and evening primrose oils.

2. Add these measured oils to a small mixing bowl and follow it up with the olive and wheatgerm oils.

3. Mix them well to combine them together and then add the blend to your pet's feed.

Essential oil blend for cuts and wounds

Oils you will need:

- 2 drops thyme oil

- 1 drop lavender oil

- 5 liters warm water

- 1 tablespoon salt

Methods of application:

1. Measure out the required oils.

2. Add the warm water to a bowl and mix in the salt.

3. Add in the oils and stir to combine them well together.

4. Wash your pet's wound in this blend.

Essential oil blend for ear infections

Oils you will need:

- 1 drop tea tree oil

- 1 drop lavender oil

- 1 drop chamomile oil

- 1 teaspoon olive oil

Methods of application:

1. Measure out the required oils.

2. Add them to a small mixing bowl and stir to combine them well together.

3. Dip a cotton ball into this blend and plug your pet's ear with it for five minutes.

Aromatherapy for your Garden

Essential Oils for the Garden

Insects	Essential Oils	Insects	Essential Oils
Ants	Spearmint, Peppermint, Citronella	Greenfly	Lavender
Aphids	Spearmint, Peppermint, Cedarwood, Hyssop	Lice	Spearmint, Peppermint Cedarwood
Bean Beetle	Thyme, Peppermint	Mosquitos	Lavender, Citronella, Lemongrass
Cabbage Rootfly	Peppermint, Sage, Rosemary, Hyssop, Thyme	Nematodes	Sage, Citronella
Carrotfly	Rosemary	Plant Lice	Spearmint, Peppermint
Caterpillars	Spearmint, Peppermint	Slugs	Cedarwood, Hyssop, Pine
Cutworm	Thyme, Sage	Snails	Cedarwood, Pine Patchouli
Flea Beetle	Peppermint, Lemongrass, Spearmint, Lavender	Ticks	Citronella, Lemongrass Thyme Sage
Fleas	Lemongrass, Citronella, Peppermint	Weevils	Cedarwood, Sandalwood, Patchouli
Flies	Lavender, Citronella, Peppermint	White Fly	Tansy, Lavender, Sage
Gnats	Spearmint, Citronella, Patchouli	Wolly Aphids	Sandalwood, Patchouli, Pine

Oils to avoid fungal growth and mold on plants

Oils you will need:

- 10 drops patchouli oil

- 10 drops cinnamon oil

- 10 drops tea tree oil

Methods of application:

1. Add any one of the above oils to your water spray dispenser.

2. Spray the plants as usual

Oils to repel insects from attacking plants

Oils you will need:

- 3 drops spearmint

- 3 drops peppermint

Methods of application:

1. Dip one of the above oils in a ball of cotton wool.

2. Place the soaked balls near your pots to repel insects such as ants, mosquitoes and slugs from attacking plants.

Conclusion

Congratulations! You now have all the information that you need to begin your journey in the world of aromatherapy. Armed with the information in this book, you should be able to combat any common issues that plague your daily life and household routines.

Remember this book acts as a basic guide to the world of aromatherapy. These chapters only scratch the surface on the means of extraction, use, therapy and even combination of oils in the areas of medication and relaxation therapy. Do not restrict yourself to the ideas and combinations in these pages alone.

With careful research, you will find more than one available solution for all the common ailments you may encounter. Most importantly, pay attention to the safety guidelines and restrictions while using these oils to ensure a safe and healthy aromatherapy experience.

Thank you for taking the time to read this book. I wish you a world of holistic, natural healing the aromatherapy way!

"No matter how big or small, acts of kindness are never wasted. With every gesture, with every step we can all make a difference in someone's life."

If you have the time to leave a positive review, it would be most gratefully appreciated.

Please check out my other books on Amazon.com (kindle and print): **Proceeds go to Charities**

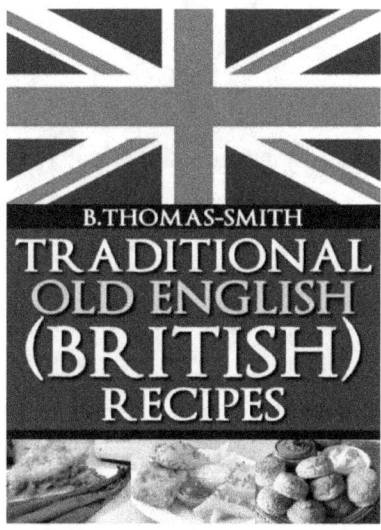

Traditional Old English Recipes on Amazon.com

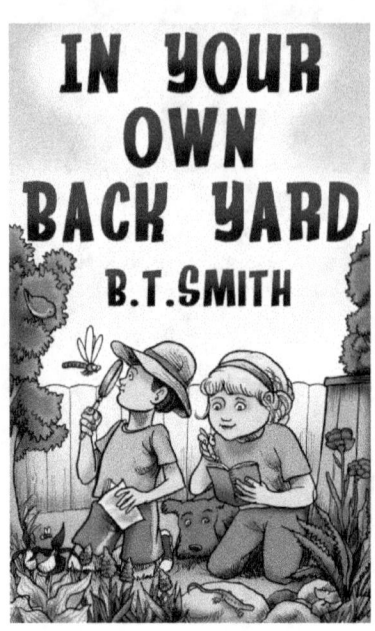

In Your Own Back Yard on Amazon.com

Thank you kindly...God Bless.